Contents

1. Foreword
1. Foreword

Nuances in cleft surgery is based on years of experience ,training and management, in the field of craniofacial and cleft surgery. My personal professional experience as a Craniofacial Orthodontist, started a few years ago in 2018 as a Fellow of the Chang Gung Memorial Hospital and direct student of Prof. Eric Liou. Chang Gung hospital is one of the most well known centers for treatment of craniofacial and cleft patients where they provide comprehensive care for the patients.

The expertise of Dr Bona Lotha, who had done both the One Year Fellowship and Six month Visiting Scholar trainings at Chang Gung Craniofacial ;served as chief plastic surgeon in Yemen Smile and later, The US Smile Train Programmes/Yemen, for seventeen years along with other consultants and mentors from Singapore (C L Yeap); Taipei Chang Gung and Childrens MA(John Mulliken), who joined him during different stages of his professional experience; are all gathered in this valuable book.

I believe that anyone who wishes to pursue a career in the field of Craniofacial and Cleft Surgery could benefit from this simplified learning guide by following the steps provided in an easy and helpful manner. I would like to personally congratulate and thank Dr. Bona Lotha for his efforts, and selfless services in the field of Craniofacial Surgery for treating many patients in Arabia and elsewhere, over the past two decades.

Best wishes to all who wish to join and serve our craniofacial and cleft angels.

Dr. Mohammad Zeinalddin
BDS; MSc; Specialty Cert: Orthodontics, M Orth FDS MFDT, Associate member of the Royal College of Surgeons of Edinburgh; Craniofacial Orthodontist fellowship CGMH Taipei
Co Founder and Board Member of the Omani Craniofacial and Cleft Society ,Muscat, Oman

Functional Aesthetic Surgery at CIHSR Department of Surgery

The Department of Surgery at CIHSR Dimapur, Nagaland offers a wide spectrum of services to the state and neighboring Indian states. Aesthetic and Reconstructive Surgery which is an integral part of the department, adds to the repertoire of treatments available to all patients.

The main focus of the Aesthetic Surgery Programme includes:

Focus on functional aesthetic surgery, which involves the correction of both appearance and function. Aesthetic Reconstructive Surgery, for deformities, trauma, post cancer reconstruction, correction of scars, and facial deformities like clefts or cancer. Many people may have a cause in appearance because of scars, and facial deformities like clefts or cancer. Many people may have a sense of dissatisfaction with appearance. This can cause immense psychosocial stress and anxiety, withdrawal and inability to express the best self.

Aesthetic surgery is not the answer to happiness in life, and is only a means to address a small part of the individual's mental health. However, the small difference could improve the person's outlook and self confidence, and we would like to make that small difference. The main aim of the aesthetic surgery programme is to bring wholesomeness to a person who has lost confidence, or the hurting individual.

Whenever possible, we try to correct deformity, enhancing the aesthetic and functional outcome, so that the person can enjoy a better quality of life, without being ostracized by society in general.

You Feel Good, when you look good

The aesthetic surgery mission of transformation can be life changing. The transformational journey after corrective aesthetic surgery is seen in one's own household

neighborhood, village and region. It can be a rewarding experience for all.

In this context, we would like to share about a novel outreach programme for cleft lip and palate children called Happy Smiles. Happy Smiles is a programme for cleft children in Nagaland and nearby states. It is all about helping underprivileged cleft patients. This is the first homegrown smile programme for cleft lip and palate children.

We have helped many underprivileged children with state of the art aesthetic reconstructive surgery, who otherwise would never have had a chance to live a normal life. Now their future looks bright, and they are confident to face the world and challenges that any normal person would undertake. As a dedicated programme for cleft patients, we offer reasonable costs for all surgeries. Patients with Ayushman cards can avail of the services. Every design we use is nuanced. However, we would advise all patients to take post-operative wound care seriously, because infections of the wound can spoil even the best of surgeries.

Dr. Temsula Alinger MS(Surgery)   Bona Lotha MS , Fellow CGMH Taipei, Board Cert AAAM Miami
HOD, Dept of Surgery   Aesthetic Craniofacial Surgeon CIHSR,
Dept. of Surgery CIHSR
Nagaland
cihsr.in

2.   Anthropometry[1] and N Vertical guide

Design the philtral flap to be

a. 2 -2.5 mm at the columellar-labial junction for a partial narrow defect *

b. 3 -4 mm between the peaks of Cupid's bow .

c. Use the full height of the cutaneous prolabium, 7 to 8 mm if available.

d. Build the median tubercle to be as plump as possible.

e. Construct the columella to be at least 4 to 5 mm in length, no longer than 7 mm.

f. Narrow the inter alar distance to be 24 mm or less.

In adults: upper philtrum width 4-4.5mm, length 14-15mm,Cupid peak to peak 8-9mm This is useful especially for secondary revision and the Abbe flap measurements

* Some prefer more than 2 mm because the width may compromise blood supply especially if the cleft is not narrow. It may be

okay for partial narrow clefts, but wider clefts may require about 3 mm above and 4.8 below

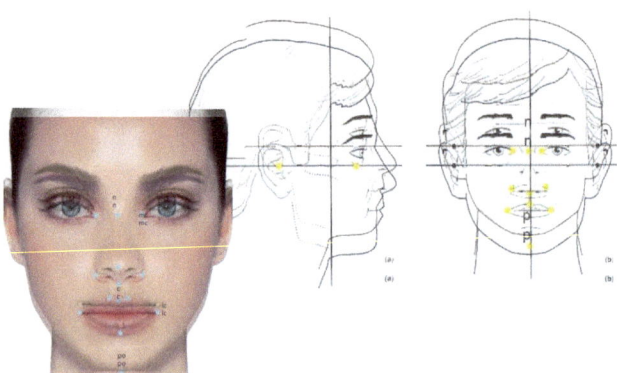

N=nasion
mc=medial canthus
c=mid Cupids point
lc=lateral commissu
pg=pogonion

The N vertical point in the natural head position helps us to
correctly align the lip and nose tissue during cleft lip repair.
The N vertical falls in line with the Centre of Cupid's bow and
Pogonion.
Any deviation from this line can be corrected during the surgery

Measurements (mm) in an adult

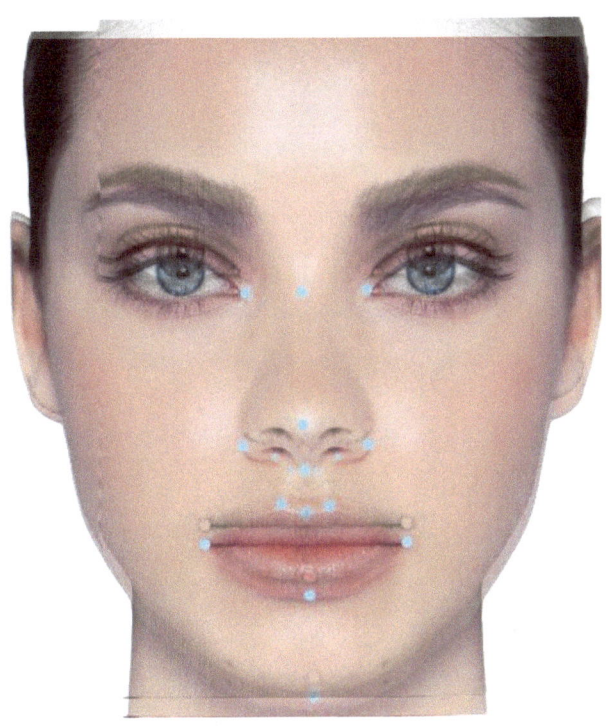

- Cupids bow
- Centre to peak 2.5
- Peak to commissure point 26
- Philtrum length 14
- Philtrum upper width 4.5
- Philtrum lower width peak to peak 8.5-9
- Alar point to Cupids peak 22
- Alar to commissure point 26
- Columella length 6-6.5
- Columella width 6-6.5
- Nostril width 6.5-7
- Nostril height 7
- Alar to alar width 31-32

3.   Nuances in unilateral cleft lip adjustments[2]

- Z plasty 1mm above Cupid white roll,on cleft side slit 2mm horizontal and fill by flap on opp side 2mm

- Red lip flap is 1mm above red white jn –

  red on red flap or at centre(earlier version)

- Incision on white roll ,slant blade to take long muscle flap

- For itf lap- note, fix cm flap and ITF to nasal mucosa

- The C flap can be used to raise the nasal sill and lengthen the columella if needed-the non cleft side is used as a guide for the nasal sill

- Muscle dissected off maxilla supra

  periosteal

- Skin incision subdermal

- Muscle closure: The 5 STEPS

  - 1. marginalis muscle

  - 2. create dimple above 1 with muscle unequal ht

  - 3.above 2 muscle lower on medial, superficial muscle derma on lateral

  - 4. muscle to col base a z plasty of muscle from cleft to non cleft side where there is a defect due to downward rotation of non cleft side muscle-this will medialize the alar base to a normal position

  - 5.subcutaneous cinch lateral ala base to opposite columella soft tissue, overcorrect

  - Tie cinching suture first,then 1 to 5

  - For Tajema- fix U flap to septal cartilage through and through

  - Use "skin hook" rule demo (OUR IDEA)

  - Ala button if needed

  - * trick in elevating philtrum is to use a muscle everting suture with a horizontal mattress suture where the U is at a deeper medial level and laterally it is more superficial with inclusion of dermis

Tajema Type 1 and Type 2 primary rhinoplasty The technique of primary rhinoplasty can be learnt in an operation theatre demonstration. Not all surgeons do primary rhinoplasty, but one can improve results if this technique is learnt.

We would like to propose two types of alar deformity for unilateral cleft lip (OUR IDEA)

1. mild deformity requiring only skin excision

2. moderate deformity requiring full reverse U incision Tajema procedure,where the alar cartilages are repositioned higher on the cleft side and domes sutured with 40 PDS

A silicon nasal conformer is used post op for 6 months after dissection of the cartilages

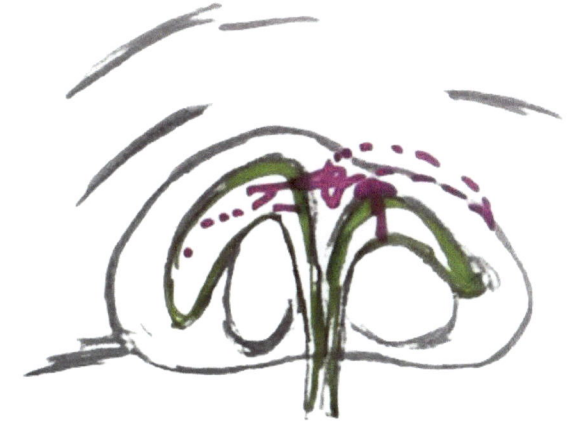

Tajima Procedure[3]
Tajima Procedure[3]

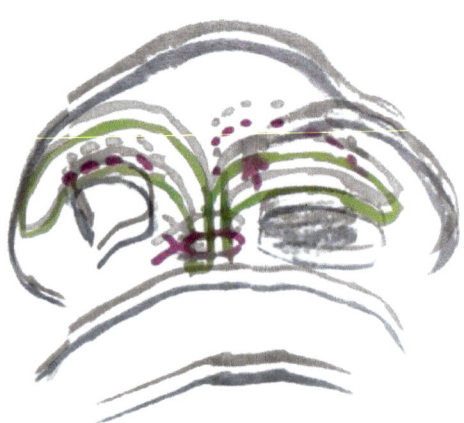

- In this procedure, we make an inverted incision over the cleft side alar skin and dissect the alar domes for some distance
- In this procedure, we make an inverted incision over the cleft side alar skin and dissect the alar domes for some distance
- The hypoplastic cleft side is overcorrected by 10-15 % via a through and through interdomal stitch with 4 0 ethilon
- The hypoplastic cleft side is overcorrected by 10-15 % via a through and through interdomal stitch with 4 0 ethilon
- The medial crura are transfixed with 4 0 vicryl
- The medial crura are transfixed with 4 0 vicryl
- Nasal conformers are used after 2 weeks for the next six months
- Nasal conformers are used after 2 weeks for the next six months

4.   **The principles and nuances of bilateral cleft lip repair[4]**
4.   **The principles and nuances of bilateral cleft lip repair[4]**

The secret of success in the field of aesthetic cleft lip surgery:
The secret of success in the field of aesthetic cleft lip surgery:

1: Symmetry
2: Primary muscle continuity
3: Proper philtral size and shape
4: Formation of the median tubercle from lateral labial elements
5: Primary positioning of the lower nasal cartilages to form the nasal tip and columella.

*J B Mulliken Current Surgical management of bilateral cleft lip in North America, Childrens Boston; PRS129:1347; 2012 June

Do not use the central lip flap

The main problem with the classical Veau technique is a whistle deformity when a central lip flap is used. The technique described here includes a few innovations:

equal lateral lip flaps are marked from A and A1at approx. 1mm above the white roll :MF are the mucosal flaps

New Cupids bow is marked at the central flap ; the measurements from the midline are roughly 4.7 mm below and about 3 mm above (as shown) the philtral pattern is cut out, 1mm above the white roll in the new
Cupid's design

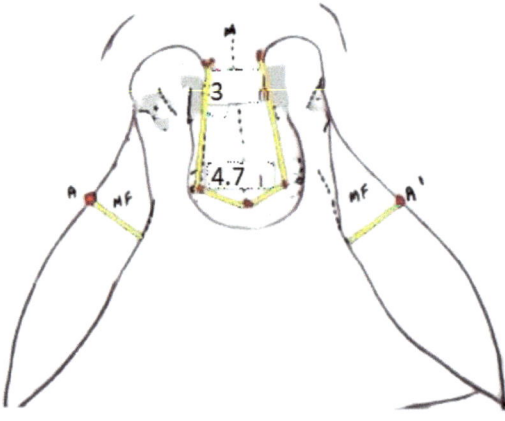

the red white line of the lip is noted as in the earlier chapter on unilateral lip; the nasal recon is also as in the earlier technique

two lateral flaps and one central flap is raised from the prolabium

the lateral prolabial flap is used for lining the buccal sulcus along with the opposite mucosal flap; like in the earlier repair the mucosal flaps are used to reconstruct the floor of nose

after final adjustments ,the lip edges are raised with a sharp blade at an angle to create the central lip flaps

The muscles are approximated in the midline, and the mucosa is closed

the central lip flaps are overcorrected by 10-15 %- this stretches post op and becomes normal later

The protuberant premaxilla is often treated pre operatively or reduced by two thumb pressure or resection during the op.

Recommended anthropometric measurements for CL in babies(Mulliken*)

Design the philtral flap to be 2 mm at the columellar-labial junction (**only in narrow clefts)

 3 mm between the peaks of Cupid's bow .

Use the full height of the cutaneous prolabium, 7 to 8 mm if available. Build the median
tubercle to be as plump as possible.

Construct the columella to be at least 4 to 5 mm in length, no longer than 7 mm. Narrow the interalar
distance to be 24 mm or less.

In adults: upper philtrum width 4-4.5mm, length 14-15mm,Cupid peak to peak 8-9mm-The measurements are useful for planning the Abbe flap

Some prefer more than 2 mm because the width may compromise blood supply especially if the cleft is not narrow. It may be okay for partial narrow clefts, but wider clefts may require about 3 mm above and 4.8 below

2006 Philip Chen original technique of bilateral lip repair
2006 Philip Chen original technique of bilateral lip repair
(Mathes 2006 July, and later Vol 3 P Neligan textbook Plastic)
(Mathes 2006 July, and later Vol 3 P Neligan textbook Plastic)

The Chang Gung bilateral cleft lip cheiloplasty technique ,Philip KT Chen,Chang Gung Memorial hospital Taipei date of operation demo: 28th March 2006

Steps:

1:markings with meth blue -bamboo tip and needle marker;prolabial markings-center1mm each side,base of col approx 2mm;triangular wings at base extend into nose;do not include mucosa in incision

2:1mm above white roll make the lateral points for the new lip

3: 2 L flaps from the lateral segments;2 prolabial flaps ,one central to cover raw area

4:no Tajima on the unilateral cleft side

5:take the measurement for appropriate silicon conformer size

Important Steps : raising the flaps
Important Steps : raising the flaps

The Prolabial skin flap is raised full thickness upto the base of the columella with lateral extensions all bleeding points are cauterized

Next, the prolabial mucosa is split into three parts-one for the central and two lateral flaps for the buccal sulcus two lateral L flaps are raised from the lateral mucosal segments.

The skin mucosa incisions start from a point 0.5-1 mm above the white roll ,extending deep into the nasal floor the inferior turbinate flaps are raised on both sides.

The muscles are dissected off the skin edges till there is no tension when the flaps are brought together formation of the nasal floor: by placing inferior turb raw surface on raw surface of L flap.

Adjust the size of the floor and then close the rest by using the prolabial lateral mucosa flap if needed an internal advancement rotation incision is made at the alar base.

Once the nasal floor is reconstructed with these flaps, attention is turned to the skin muscle, mucosa flap.

Important steps: the philtrum, muscle flaps and median tubercle

Formation of the Philtrum

The lower part of the flap includes two through and through sutures as: Muscle mucosa on one side to mucosa muscle same distance on

other side , and then from this side mucosa-opposite side mucosa and muscle.

The upper end below the buccal sulcus is only mucosa.

The subcutaneous edges are approximated till there is no tension at all on the flaps

 Next, the prolabial flap is made to sit on this midline defect and approximated with the two lateral lip mucosal flaps which have been raised from the lip edges.

The midline of the lip should be reconstructed in such a way that there appears a definite "pout" of the central region close the vermillion with

everted horizontal sutures to increase lip pout.

The rest of the mucosa is then closed.

The repaired lip may look somewhat tight in appearance and bulging at the center-this is done intentionally because the lip will be

stretched to a more normal position post op over the next few weeks and months.

Since there is no central mucosal flap like in the earlier Veau design,patients do not develop a whistle deformity.

Any excess in the lateral wings is trimmed off and the two sides of the repaired nasal floor and ala base are compared for size and symmetry. Some surgeons like to

cinch the alar region and also cinch the naso labial and NLF in wider clefts;this is optional, and many do not use it.

Important steps: Primary Rhinoplasty

Tajima:

The Tajima alar incisions are made and the cartilages dissected from under the skin the alar cartilages

are overcorrected 20%.

A transfixation PDS stitch is passed through the medial crura after the Tajima flaps are sutured together by passing the needle from one end to the other over the alar cart to make a U turn across the flaps.

Two internal PDS buttons are placed to shape the alar region post op:

After the wound heals, use a conformer for 6mths to retain the shape of the alar cart and also to maintain the columella

length.

Modifying the Nuances at Happy Smiles CIHSR

- In the CIHSR modified Tajima, a through and through cartilaginous suture is used only for bulbous tips or when columella elongation is needed. Otherwise, the suture passes superficial to the domes and only medial transfixation is used for the medial plates. Some overcorrection is achieved, and after two weeks a 3D printed nasal conformer is used for six months.

- The marginalis muscle is hitched to the dermis of the philtral flap to enhance the "dip" in philtrum

- The lateral philtral escarpments are enhanced by suturing the lateral edge at a higher level. This raises the philtral edge[5].

- We create a Parisian pout of the median tubercle area by dissecting off mucosa for approx. 1mm and using everting horizontal mattress sutures.

- An internal nasal cinch is used with 3 0 proline or nylon. This corrects alar flaring. Nylon is better than proline, because proline tends to have suture memory and may loosen later.

- Horizontal mattress sutures are used to approximate the peripheralis. Additional alar buttoning is done with 3 0 nylon or proline

- In our case last week for an 11 year old BCCL, we have changed some of the anthropometric nuances to keep the measurements between the 8 and adult measurements. This gives a more balanced look. The upper philtral width was kept at 4mm and lower at 6mm, length between 12-1? mm, and angle of Cupid from peak to centre at approx. 30 degrees. Columella length at approx. 6-6.5mm

- The incision for lateral lip elements was 1mm above the white roll. Unlike the Black technique, no prolabial mucosa is used. Instead, the marking are 1mm above the white roll.

Changes made at Surgery, CIHSR design
Changes made at Surgery, CIHSR design

- For floor of nose, we reserve the inferior turbinate for future use if needed, and use only lone L and M tailored flaps. An adequate buccal sulcus is also designed.

- Steristrips are recommended for six months post op, No tension repair because of long muscle flaps and no Botox needed.

- Massage therapy post op is quite helpful. In some cases of Type 3-4 Fitzpatrick sun types, we suggest low dose triamcinolone for the scar, derma pen needling, pico laser and tyrosinase inhibitors.

- We avoid the lateral triangular fork flaps in our cases. We are able to get an adequate gain in columella length without these flaps.

- If needed, in a long lip, we add a small muscle hitch to caudal septum to prevent a long lip.

- The interface of aesthetic medicine and plastic surgery helps one plan better outcomes in such cases, especially the older cleft patient, where surgery is more complicated.

- This is useful for the median tubercle enhancement, since the median tubercle tends to lag behind the increase in philtral width post operatively.

- We would need to study the older cleft patients because so far there is no data on this concept of philtral widening or median tubercle lag in older patients.

- An FEM (finite element motion) study could be useful for this change

6. Sessions with Mulliken on bilateral clefts and Tessier 7

Dear John,

A consultant craniofacial surgeon from Tokyo has some interesting questions on bil cleft lip terms. Please could you advise us on this?

Thanks again, bona TOKYO:

"Today, I would like to ask you of a technical term about cleft lip. Many article described drawing line as curvilinear line or concave line. As you know, Dr. Mulliken also use the term "biconcave line" in bilateral cleft lip design.

But some Japanese surgeon use the term of "convex line" when they explain curvilinear line. Is it common technical term in your community or your mentor, Dr. Mulliken?this is personal question.I hope to have your professional comment about that.

warm regards,
Nobuhiro Sato.

Hi Bona,

The word *curvilinear* (from Latin) simply means "curved line" or

bounded by curved lines. Maybe this explains why Japanese

use *convex line* for *curvilinear line*. The terms *convex* and *concave* in English to describe a curvilinear shape, but one has to be certain from which perspective on the shape is determined.

My serial measurements of philtral scars in BCCL demonstrate how cphs-cphs and cphi-cphi differentially widen with growth. See Kim D.C., Mulliken J.B. *Plast.Reconstr. Surg.* 2017;140:326e.

If the philtral incisions are designed straight or biconvex, the philtral shape widens superiorly more than inferiorly. Therefore, I recommend that the philtral incisions b drawn initially in
a *biconcave* shape and more narrow at the columellar-labial junction.

 I hope this explanation is clear…

John Mulliken, Childrens MA

Re: repair tranverse oral cleft[6] , Dr Temsula team @ CIHSR Surgery Dept, Nagaland

Treatment of lateral cleft lip,with Mulliken JB.

Child with Tessier 7 @ CIHSR Surgery Dept, for online video demo July

21, 2021 Pandemic surgery online

Hi John,

This Tessier 7 at CIHSR for online adv as they plan to operate.

1. don't think the Korean paper idea of z plasty or geometric incisions is a good idea at all for Type 3-6 Fitzpatrick skin types..bad scarring later

2. suggest simple linear closure with fine nylon and steristrips

muscle overlapping not needed; enough to use 4 0 vicryl. There is no great advantage

3. the idea of overcorrection, though arbitrary is useful. I mm shorter on cleft side makes sense due to

some stretching post op Hi Bona, Agree Z-plasty is wrong. Also prefer vermilion-commissure flap at

commissure rather than butt-joint closure.

Best,

John

Childrens Boston MA

Bon Chance for surgery next week, Dr Temsula and team,.. Christian Referral Hospital Surgery, Dimapur Nagaland..unfortunately i can't do the demo..am in Noida city, resting and clearing the clutter in my brain!

 Yes, the inferiorly based rectangular vermilion mucosal flap is a great idea, along with closure of the orbicularis oris muscle sling as a counterforce to the contraction of the cutaneous scar,as you taught! No butt-joint stuff...haha

8:Variations on floor of nose reconstruction

Using

1: The inferior turbinate flap with mucosal flaps[7]

2: No inferior turbinate flap; only mucosal flaps

To adjust the nasal floor:

a: An inferior turbinate flap I(pear) is raised by extending an incision from the mucosa at the edge of the alveolus upto the superior base of the inferior turbinate; from here an inferior flap is raised which is about 2cm long; at the superior edge of the info turbinate a small intercartilagenous incision about 0.5 cm is made transversely; all fibrous attachments to at the base are released and complete homeostasis secured because this is the site which causes troublesome bleeding post op

The inferior turbinate flap is rotated into the pyriform rim defect and sutured; next the lateral L shaped buccal flap is raised from the level of the skin for a short distance without including the mucosa over the alveolus and folded on itself to fill the defect lateral to the inf turbinate flap in the pyriform area

This buccal flap is next folded over itself and joined to the opposite mucosal flap from the edge of the cleft side to bridge the gap formed by the cleft

Finally; the skin edges are trimmed and brought together to design the nasal floor:

11: Remove excess tissue in between; a figure of 8 stitch is placed on the lip muscle:the Z plasty is completed; sometimes a cheiloplasty de la croix is placed in the undersurface mucosa; two alar button sutures are placed to treat the alar dead space:

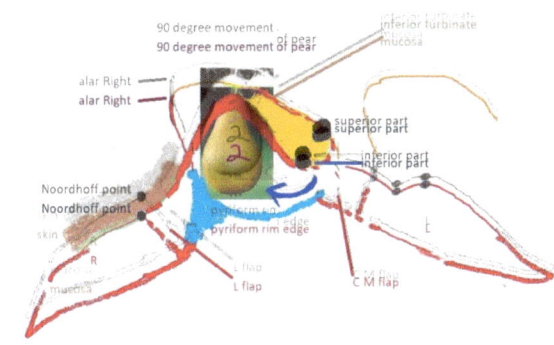

Fig: Analogy of the pear

23

Putting the three flaps together to reconstruct the floor of nose using the analogy of a pear (OUR IDEA)

Imagine the inferior turbinate is like a pear handing inside the nostril tree

The incisional approach to the inferior
pole of the
inferior turbinate flap is easy-
trace along the Noordhoff point
and incise between skin and
mucosa up the vestibule and cut
along the inferior part of the
turbinate-just follow the pear all
around and connect to the
superior pole.
A small transverse stab between the
lower lateral cartilages is the superior
entry point.
Connect the pear and after removing
the bone to prevent curling of the
flap,rotate it down by 90 degrees.

The superior pole edge is fixed to
the pyriform edge to provide lining
for the nose.

Pyriform rim

inferior turbinate mucosa

90 degree movement of pear

alar Right

superior part

inferior part

Noordhoff point

pyriform rim edge

skin

R

L

mucosa

L flap

C M flap

The inferior edge joins the L flap and is sutured as

a turn over flap to the turned over CM flap.

This completes the floor of nose correction.

Floor of nose recon using only two mucosal flap modification at Hap by Smiles CIHSR, Dept of Surge
Floor of nose recon using only two mucosal flap modification at Happy Smiles CIHSR, Dept of Surge

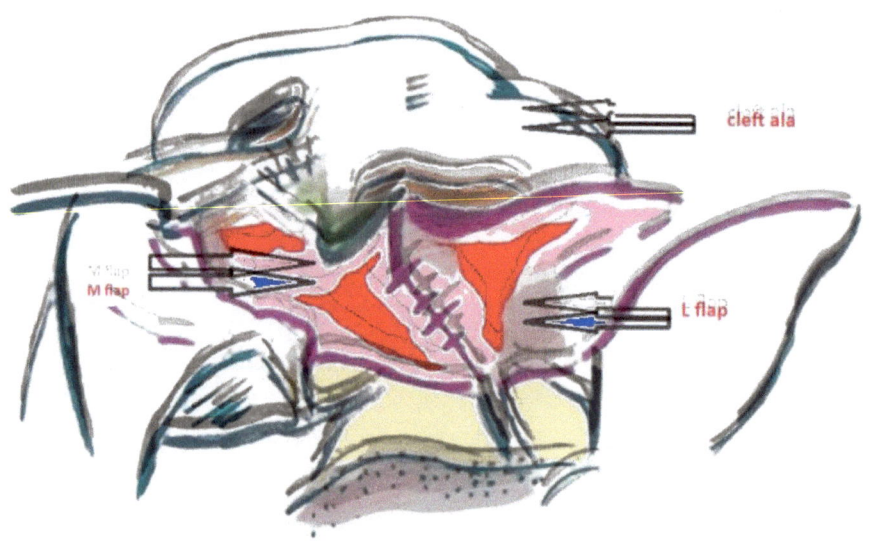

The Cleft Palate-Craniofacial Journal 2020, Vol. 57(4S) 1-143 ª 2020, American Cleft Palate-Craniofacial Association

Article reuse guidelines: sagepub.com/journals-permissions DOI: 10.1177/1055665620901804 journals.sagepub.com/home/cpc

Abstract no 17: Anatomy of the KISS Principle for Trainee Cleft Surgeons: The Quest for a Cleft Aesthetic Code of the Philtrum and Median Tubercle in Unilateral Cleft Lip Surgery

Background/Purpose:

Methods/Description:

Results: A successful repair of a cleft lip deformity includes proper alignment of all the labial and alar elements, floor of nose reconstruction when needed, adequate muscle flaps for symmetric closure, and a dynamic philtrum as well as an attractive pout of the median tubercle.

Conclusions: Getting it right the first time is an important aspect of cleft lip surgery. Understanding the nuances of a cleft lip surgery requires experience with large numbers of surgeries, because no 2 cleft lip deformities are the same. There are many good techniques and plastic surgeons have personal preferences, but the most important variable in the successful repair of a cleft lip deformity includes proper alignment of all the labial and alar elements, floor of nose reconstruction when needed, adequate muscle flaps for symmetric closure, and a dynamic philtrum as well as an attractive pout of the median tubercle.

9: Nuances of Cleft Palate Surgery

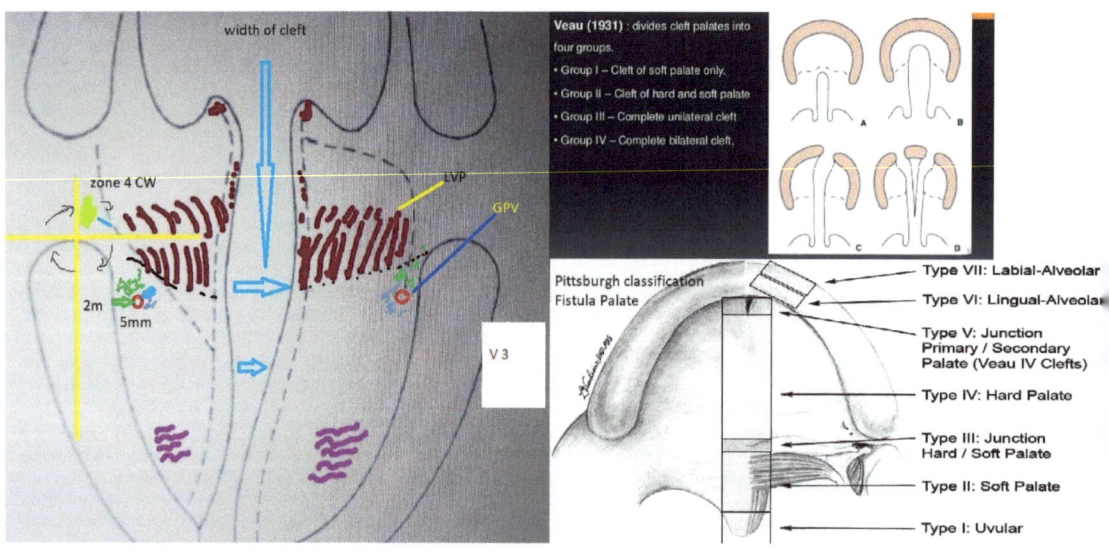

width of cleft

zone 4 CW

LVP

GPV

2m

5mm

V 3

Veau (1931) : divides cleft palates into
four groups.
• Group I – Cleft of soft palate only.
• Group II – Cleft of hard and soft palate
• Group III – Complete unilateral cleft
• Group IV – Complete bilateral cleft,

Pittsburgh classification
Fistula Palate

Type VII: Labial-Alveolar

Type VI: Lingual-Alveolar

Type V: Junction
Primary / Secondary
Palate (Veau IV Clefts)

Type IV: Hard Palate

Type III: Junction
Hard / Soft Palate

Type II: Soft Palate

Type I: Uvular

Nuances: Anatomical considerations in cleft palate surgery Modified technique

1. The levator sling is created : the muscles are detached from their abnormal insertions on the palatal bone and retro positioned to make them meet in the midline at a distance of 7-10mm (this step is not needed if a double opposing z plasty is used)

2. A button hole incision below the middle of the maxillary tuberosity identifies the Hamulus which is fractured to medialize the muscle complex

3. The tensor tendon is incised as it hooks around the Hamulus process of the sphenoid bone

4. The palatal aponeurosis formed by the levator and tensor, insert on the posterior surface of the palatal bone; this is incised with a sharp blade to release the muscle fully

5. the elevation of hard palate mucoperiosteum is made in the middle zone near the palatal rugae,where the attachment is looser.

6. The neuro vascular bundle lies about 5mm mm medial to the 2ndmolar –care is taken to dissect this structure so that the flap can be moved easily to the midline

7. The lateral raw surface is filled with buccal fat or surgicel

8. A 5 mm double opposing z plasty is made at the lower end of the soft palate

9. The uvularis muscle is well approximated

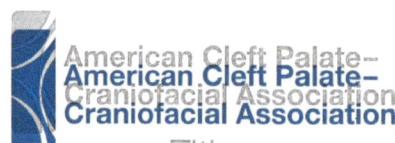

American Cleft Palate–
Craniofacial Association

Title
Rules of engagement in minimal blood loss palatoplasty using saline hydro dissection: a useful learning curve for younger cleft surgeons in maneuvering areas of static resistance due to tight tissue planes

Date : April 29, 2021

Presenter: Bona Lotha, Primary Cleft Surgeon
Yemen Global Smiles and Smile Train Programmes ,Sanaa Yemen
Title : Mr

disclosures

- No disclosures

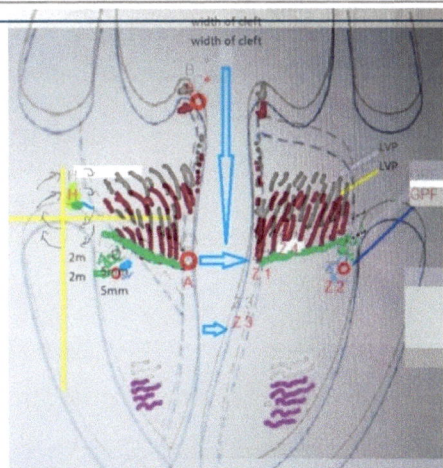

Figure 17: Areas of "static resistance" in cleft palate surgery, due to tight tissue planes.

H-position of hamulus
LVP- levators
GPF- greater palatine foramen, in children, 5mm from maxillary molars 2-3
Static Resistance Zones
Z1- posterior spine area
Z2- GPF area
Z3- Nasal mucosa area hard palate
Z4- aponeurosis
soft palate length- 12-18mm in children, 37+/-4mm in adults

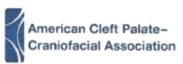
American Cleft Palate–
Craniofacial Association

Innovations

- Minimal blood loss in palatoplasty can be achieved with the simple 1997 Haifa concept of adrenaline saline hydrodissection
- and,
- a good knowledge of key anatomical structures, as well as the stubborn areas of static resistance, where dissection is difficult because of fixed tissue planes

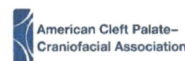
American Cleft Palate–
Craniofacial Association

Zones of static resistance

- Palate dissection can get messy for younger cleft surgeons who are learning to identify the difficult areas of tissue resistance, especially during overseas assignments.

- Identifying key areas in palatoplasty helps the cleft surgeon avoid intraoperative complications, and also reduces blood loss

- Some of the key areas we have mentioned above include the position of hamulus, greater palatine foramen, the area around the posterior spine, medial edge of the hard palate, mid rugae of the palate, the palatal aponeurosis and the sagittal inclination of the levators in cleft palate.

Thank you

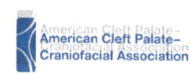

- The learning curve is reasonable and techniques can be added, as one gains more experience with cleft palate surgeries.

Techniques of palatoplasty for complete cleft palate (   )
Techniques of palatoplasty for complete cleft palate (MODIFIED)

Position of patient
Position of patient
Rose position with hyperextension of the neck, by placing a roll under the neck
Rose position with hyperextension of the neck, by placing a roll under the neck

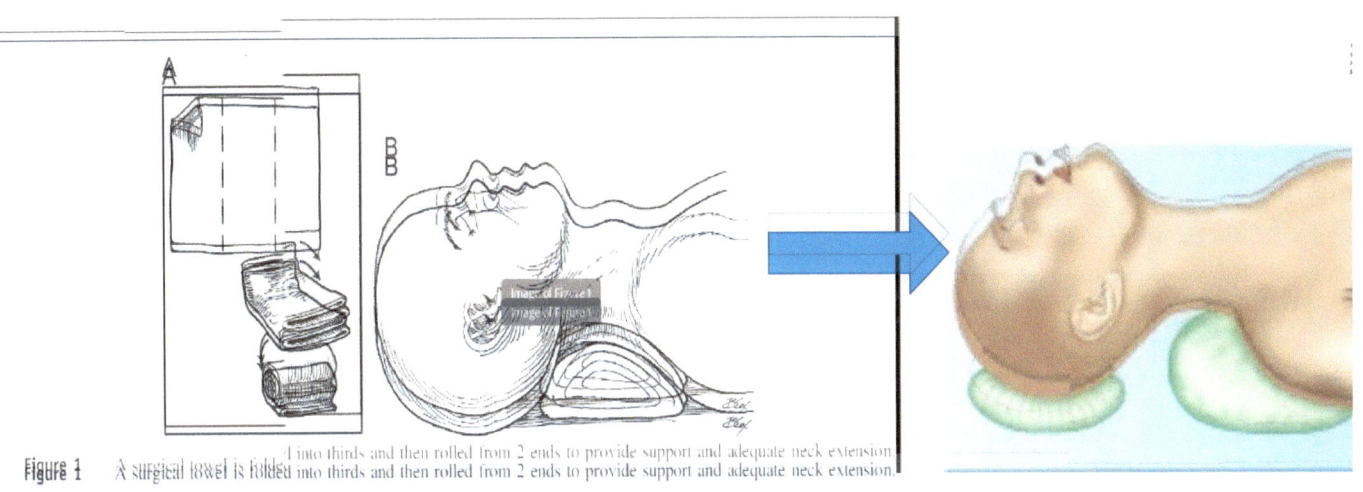

Figure 1 A surgical towel is folded into thirds and then rolled from 2 ends to provide support and adequate neck extension.

A surgical towel is folded into thirds and then rolled from 2 ends to provide support and adequate neck extension.

2012 minimal incision palatoplasty with levator repositioning

In this method, we use a relatively bloodless minimal incision method using 1:500,000 saline adrenaline hyrdrodissection[8] by mixing 1mg adrenaline in 500 ml saline

Starting from the medial minimal incisions,using fine curved sharp scissors, the levators are dissected from their insertion on

the palatal aponeurosis / bony hard palate

Repositioning of the muscles in a transverse position; the uvular is 2/3 retro positioned

a small button hole incision is added in Zone 4, over the hamulus to fracture the bone, incise the tensor and medialize the muscles.

The surgery takes 20-25 minutes, and is very safe

The complete palate is closed in 2 stages- stage one includes soft palate closure with levator repositioning; the stage 2

minimal incision palatoplasty is done after 6 months to a year

No intra/ post op bleeds or hypoxia in any case The

levator repositioning improves speech

The nasal flaps are best approached from the lateral side to prevent tearing ;the undersurface is dissected with a fine elevator in a gentle, horizontal direction

It is best to raise the mucoperiosteal flaps from the mid palate where the tissue is loose and less vascular Palatal fistula is usually due

to wrong technique and too much tension on the flaps and ,wound infection,

Two flap palatoplasty[9] incision markings

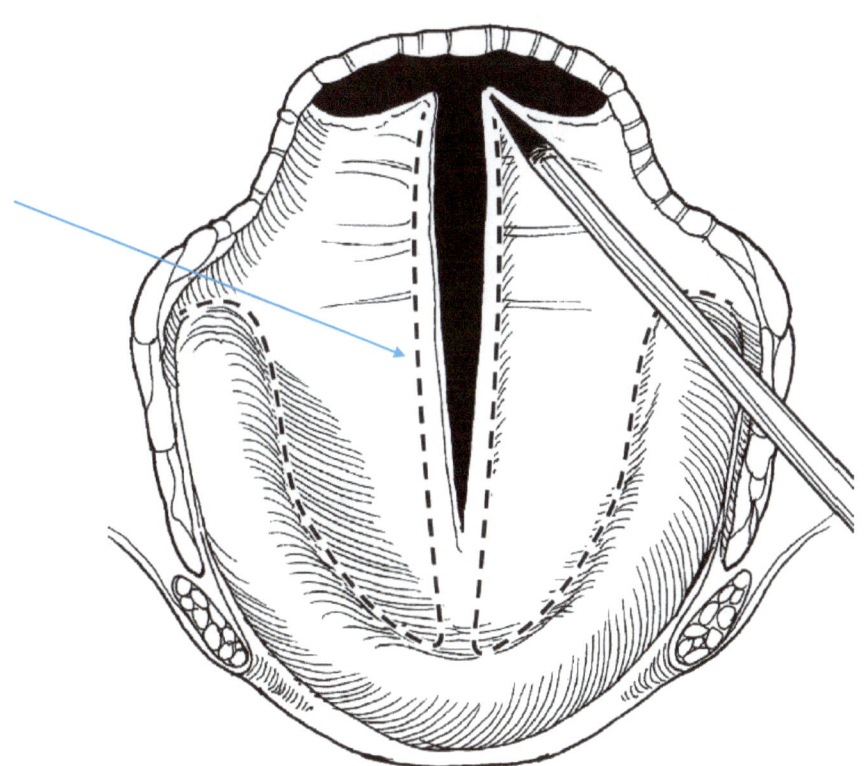

Keep adequate tissue on
nasal side for closure

The nasal flap is dissected
horizontally, and not in an inferior
direction. This prevents holes.

Figure 2   Outline of the proposed incision for a 2-flap palatoplasty.

Anatomy of GPV and Levators

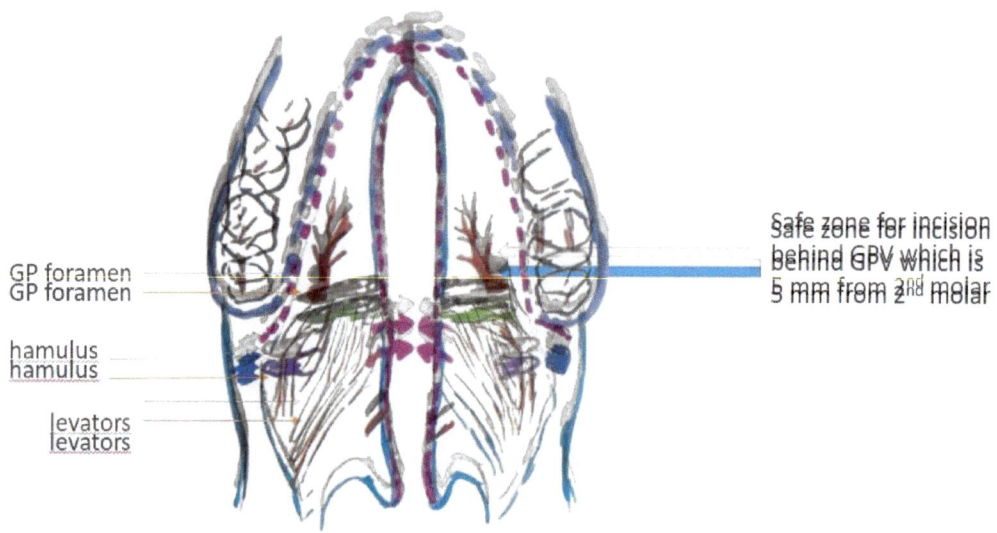

GP foramen
GP foramen

hamulus
hamulus

levators
levators

Safe zone for incision behind GPV which is 5 mm from 2nd molar

SOFT PALATE

45 degree double opposing z plasty anterior and
posterior 5mm flaps
45 degree double opposing z plasty anterior and
Cinch with 4 0 vicryl closure
posterior 5mm flaps
* Cinch with 4 0 vicryl after closure

Left incision in   includes the
mucosa and muscle Leave some
Left incision in RED includes the
muscle on posterior mucosa
mucosa and muscle Leave some
muscle on posterior mucosa

The   incision on the left is
mucosa with a bit of muscle on it to
The Green incision on the left is
provide support
mucosa with a bit of muscle on it to
provide support

Right incision in   includes
only mucosa
Right incision in RED includes
only mucosa
The Green incision includes
muscle and mucosa
The Green incision includes
muscle and mucosa

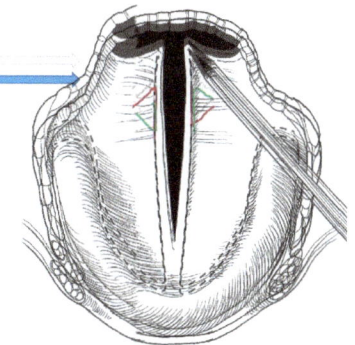

Steps in releasing attachments

Tips in cleft palate techniques

- Dissection of the abnormal attachments of the velar musculature and retro positioning to create a functional sling is key and must be performed in all clefts regardless of severity
- the mucoperiosteal flaps are elevated starting at the lateral edges and proceeding to the cleft edge to ensure there is adequate mucosa for closure of the nasal lining before incising the edge of the cleft hard palate
- in dissecting the uvula, most of the tissue is left on the nasal side and closed with mattress sutures; this creates a bulky pad and enhances the contact between the velum and the posterior pharyngeal wall, contributing to velopharyngeal closure
- the neurovascular bundle is mobilized to improve the mobility of the mucoperiosteal flap-the cone of periosteum at the base of the bundle is incised with a fine blade and two parallel incisions are made 2mm from the bundle-a right angled forceps loosens the bundle

Further mobilization of the flaps

This step is not
needed in double
opposing z plasty

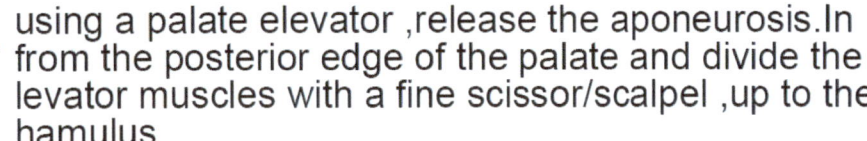

- using a palate elevator ,release the aponeurosis.In from the posterior edge of the palate and divide the levator muscles with a fine scissor/scalpel ,up to the hamulus
- incise the tendon of the tensor as it hooks around the hamulus-this facilitates the medial mobilization of the muscle complex
- the anterior vomer flap ,starting at the anterior edge of the cleft and extending to the junction of the hard and soft palate ,is used in almost all cases to close the nasal lining-this minimizes tension and less oral mucosa needs to be turned in for the lining
- Never transact the nasal mucosa (Onizuka) because it leads to scarring

Double opposing z plasty[10] for the soft palate

Linear closure of the soft palate leads to scarring and shortening and worsening of VPI The levator muscle occupy the lower 40% of the soft palate

A double opposing z plasty is designed to lengthen the palate by a few cm

The uvularis muscle is approximated since it also contributes to speech improvement

The raw lateral surface after repair
The raw lateral surface after repair

The raw lateral surfaces are lined with buccal fat to prevent any post operative pain; surgicel is also used for hemostasis

The buccal fat is approached via a stab incision a few mm above the retro molar mucosa, and using scissors, the buccinators fascia is opened. This leads to prolapse of the fat which is then gently teased out using two non tooth forceps- the first gently pulls out the fat which is held by the 2nd pair of forceps. The process is repeated till an adequate length is released.

Hammock 4-0 Vicryl sutures are used to fix the fat to the repair so that the buccal fat does not prolapse into the oral cavity

If the nuances are followed ,there should be minimal bleeding even in a complete palatoplasty procedure.

10. What's New in Cleft Surgery in 2024?

Not just designing cleft repairs, but also, finally creating one's own cleft lip defect for helping post trauma patients!

In November 2023, after many years of designing cleft lip repairs, A NEW CHALLENGE!

An adult Vietnamese male patient presented with a post traumatic scar of the upper lip (fig) at the OMS Hospital, Ho Chi Min City, Vietnam. The surgeons sent the photos to our unit at CIHSR, Nagaland, last week for a possible solution. We had never seen such a case before and so traced the defect and decided to create a cleft lip defect with a long muscle flap, and larger z skin flaps along with C flap to address the short lip and vermillion excess. Dr P Uy and his team operated the patient this week with good outcomes. Some minor revisions will be needed in the future.(picture in last section)

This is the first case report in the world for creating a cleft lip defect to address a post traumatic scar. There are several technical challenges in such large defects, but following the nuances of cleft lip repair, one is able to get a fairly good outcome. Since the muscle dictates the skin movement in cleft lip surgery, we focused on a long muscle flap, followed by z flaps of the skin. The result of such a combination allows for lengthening of the philtrum and a reasonably good looking lip.

11. Suggested Reading

1. Direct Anthropometry of Repaired Bilateral Complete Cleft Lip: A Long-Term Assessment ,D Kim and Mulliken, Plastic and Reconstructive Surgery June 2014 Volume 140, Number 2

2. Chang Gung Technique of Unilateral Cleft Lip Repair , Philip Kuo-Ting Chen,Craniofacial Center, Chang Gung Memorial Hospital, Taipei, Taiwan, China, Cleft Lipp and Palate primary repair, Sommerlad and Bing, Springer

3. Chang Gung Technique of Bilateral Cleft Lip Repair, Philip Kuo-Ting Chen ,Craniofacial Center, Chang Gung Memorial Hospital, Taipei, Taiwan, China, Sommerlad and Bing, Springer 2013

4. Current Surgical management of bilateral cleft lip in North America, J B Mulliken ,Childrens Boston, PRS129:1347, 2012 June

5. The Philtrum in Cleft Lip: Review of Anatomy and Techniques for Construction Carolyn Rogers, Mulliken et al, The Journal of Craniofacial Surgery & Volume 25, Number 1, January 2014

6. Treatment of lateral cleft lip,Rogers, GF, Mulliken JB. PRS 2007;120:728.

7. Learning to Crack the Cleft Aesthetic Code in Unilateral Cleft Lip Surgery by Younger Cleft Trainees: Using Nuances and the Innovative Taipei Pear Analogy for Inferior Turbinate-flap Floor of Nose Reconstruction Lotha B, Bergonzani and Zeinalddin M, *Acta Scientific Paediatrics* 3.9 (2020): 10-16.

Suggested reading
Suggested reading

8: Intraoperative expansion of the palate by the tumescent technique(Ideas and Innovations) , Issac J et al, Haifa Israel,PRS vol: 100:1 July 1997

9: Rules of Engagement in Minimal Blood Loss Palatoplasty Using Saline Hydro Dissection: A Useful Learning Curve for Younger Cleft Surgeons in Maneuvering Areas of Static Resistance due to Tight Tissue Planes, Lotha B and Mohd Z *Acta Scientific Medical Sciences* 4.11 (2020): 36-42.

10: Cleft palate repair by double opposing z plasty: LT Furlow:Op Tech in Plastic Surgery 2:4 223-232 1995

Acknowledgments of mentors over the years
Acknowledgments of mentors over the years

1: John Mulliken, Childrens MA, lifetime mentor for the incredible lessons over many years
1: John Mulliken, Childrens MA, lifetime mentor for the incredible lessons over many years

2: Chang Gung Craniofacial Centre, Taipei for the excellent training over several years
2: Chang Gung Craniofacial Centre, Taipei for the excellent training over several years

3: CL Yeap, Cosmetic and Plastic Surgery, Mount Elizabeth Singapore, for all the aesthetic surgery lessons over many years
3: CL Yeap, Cosmetic and Plastic Surgery, Mount Elizabeth Singapore, for all the aesthetic surgery lessons over many years

Lesson Videos

In addition top reading materials on unilateral cleft,bilateral cleft lip,and palatoplasty ,please refer to the videos supplied for

1. UCL Philip Chen Taipei Chang Gung

2. BCL Philip Chen Taipei Chang Gung

3. Palatoplasty LJ Lo Taipei Chang Gung

Available for ref at our google classroom series(For classroom CODE, mail: docbonalotha@gmail.com) Related papers by our group

in Muscat, Oman online: https://aestheticmedplastcraniofacial.wordpress.com/

Remarks: Cleft surgery is best learnt during operation theatre demonstrations by an experienced cleft surgeon. You are encouraged to learn the fine aspects of primary lip, primary rhinoplasty and palate surgery before proceeding further in cleft surgery

Learning to analyze important journal papers

with

John Mulliken

Cleft Lip Nasal Deformity: Foundation-Based Approach to Primary Rhinoplasty R Tse et al PRS Nov 2019
Discussions with John B Mulliken Childrens MA Nov 2019 Mulliken, John Tue, 12 Nov, 22:31

Unilateral Cleft Lip Nasal Deformity: Foundation-Based Approach to Primary Rhinoplasty, R Tse et al PRS Nov 2019

Bona;

I just submitted a paper to PRS: long-term study of nasal revision in100 patients with UCCL (Yao CA and Mulliken JB). She found only 13% never needed revision; about 65% needed 2 or more. Furthermore, "transfixion sutures" required more revisions than semi-open inter cartilaginous sutures. If you want to spin your head around, read Nov. PRS article, pg. 1138: Tse RW, et al. claim that nasal deformity is corrected by straightening columella and correcting the nasal floor and sidewall-- without tip dissection! Only 2 revisions need at age 5 years (n=102). This is Fisher concept of postponing nasal correction. If you have time to read the article, I'd be interested in your opinion. My reading, observation, and understanding is that the unilateral cleft lip nasal deformity is a difficult problem; not so easily solved at primary repair.

John

Dear John;

Thanks for sharing this paper. First of all, I would like to say that the concepts presented are really, mostly a mix of Noordhoff and Tord Skoog; and several others ; the "Fisher technique" ;in all fairness to great pioneers, is taken from Noordhoff's Chang Gung cheiloplasty and it's many revisions over 40 odd years. There is nothing unique or "NEW" in this reinvention of the cleft wheel, but rather a description of old wine in new wineskins, including some advanced tech. I read the paper, thinking to myself: This is what great pioneers like Skoog,Noordhoff,Mulliken and others have been doing for so many years… I personally like new ideas; but having read quite a bit on the evolution of technique since Rose Thompson 1890s and Skoog, I think there is "nothing new under the cleft sun" in this day and age;although innovations on older techniques happen on a regular basis without any consensus between cleft surgeons worldwide. I have excerpts from the paper with my comments in red:

Best;

Bona

Childrens Hospital MA Discussions
Childrens Hospital MA Discussions

- unilateral cleft lip nasal deformity results
- from displacement of underlying base elements1
- and consequent collapse of the arch
- forms that define the nose

- *comment: using this as a basis for their hypothesis , but should have mentioned the different types of tip deformities in cleft children that give one an idea about whether or not tip procedures are absolutely necessary.. eg. Asian.Latino,African tips etc.. Are very different from Caucasians . I don't not think tip procedures are always needed, but one cannot use the one shoe fits all approach*

- primary
- rhinoplasty involving nasal tip dissection is often
- performed, recurrent deformity is common;
  and
- secondary correction is undertaken in 35 to 74
- percent of patients

- *comment: interesting, because one always wondered why there was so much focus on "tip surgery" ;sometimes it is not necessary*

  ,but it does not mean one has to do away with this procedure

51

- no nasal tip dissection
- can be performed at the same time, adequate
- correction may be achieved by work on the underlying
- "foundation" alone
- *Comment:* No nasal tip… what type of tip needs tip procedures? Obviously, not all and so one needs to clarify this. What about a thick bulbous tip seen in quite a few?

- For lateral wall advancement, mucoperiosteum
- within the nasal cavity is raised and
- incision is taken along the cleft margin with a vertical
- back cut. The flap is advanced en bloc with
- the alar base so that mucoperiosteum spans the
- gap between piriform aperture and the new alar
- base position.
- *Comment:* credit goes to Tord Skoog for this idea, but not many takers here on this technique. Some in Europe argue you get off bone formation, others not so eager because results vary and may not be useful

Childrens Hospital MA Discussions

- For turbinate flap, vertical release along the
- piriform aperture is made up to the base of the
- turbinate so that the anteriorly based flap fills the
- defect. The L-flap is based on mucoperiosteum,
- with an incision continued along the cleft margin
- to allow closure of the nasal floor.
- *Comment: Noordhoff's L flap(using Millard idea) is not used commonly these days because modifications on the inferior turbinate flap at CGMH by his disciples have replaced his earlier techniques. Altogether, there are nearly 4-5 modifications, each technique is a reinvention of that "same cup of tea": not too much to add really*

- Subperiosteal septoplasty. The anterior nasal spine and septum are accessed by
- means of the medial lip incision (*below, left*). Transverse incision through premaxillary
- periosteum (*solid green line*) provides access for subperiosteal dissection on either side
- of the anterior nasal spine and eventually under the septum. Release of periosteum on
- the noncleft side (*blue dotted line*) allows the septum to reposition to the midline of
- the face
- *comment: Court Cutting is no believer in the ANS..controversial. As for caudal septum procedures, many use different variations for repositioning and this is commonly used by some in Taiwan and other countries*

53

Childrens Hospital MA Discussions

Childrens Hospital MA Discussions

- Nasal tip dissection is not performed. Septoplasty,
- alar advancement, lateral sidewall reconstruction,
- and floor closure produce the majority
- of the nasal correction..
- comment: *used by some, others prefer variations*

- A transfixion suture through the "empty triangle"
- is used to exclude muscle lateral to the
- ala and to adhere vestibular mucosa to skin
- along the alar crease. Additional alar transfixion
- sutures are used to obliterate the vestibular
- web and accentuate the alar crease.
- Comment: *muscle z plasties are commonly used by many, and web procedures not always favored because not long lasting*

Childrens Hospital MA Discussions

- Columellar
- angle, nostril width ratio, and lateral lip height
- ratio have been found to be the most important
- anthropometric indices of the unilateral cleft
- lip nasal deformity
- comment: *commonly used by many*

- a vertical back-cut
- (*green*) toward the base of the inferior turbinate: lateral nasal wall is advanced en bloc with the alar base (*center, right*) so that mucoperiosteum spans the piriform aperture and the new anterior position of alar base donor site along the bony wall is left to reepithelialize. The nasal floor is closed by approximating the flap to septal mucosa :: Nasal floor closure: Mucoperiosteum is inset into septal mucosa from posterior to anterior.
- *Comment:* the inferior turbinate flap techniques vary, but some avoid it because of post operative bleeding from the raw surface and prefer mucosal flaps. A matter of preference
- *TYPE* of cleft lip defect narrow to moderate width cleft lip defect : important in decision making

Childrens Hospital MA Discussions

- **Turbinate versus L-Flap versus Lateral Wall**
- **Advancement**
- Among patients with complete clefts that had
- 5-year follow-up, five, eight, and four underwent
- L-flap, turbinate flap, and lateral wall advancement,
- respectively…late postoperative period, L-flap was associated with better columellar angle, whereas lateral nasal flap was associated with better lateral lip height ratio
- Comment: *Noordhoff's group use variations every week..last 40 plus years*

- **Alveolar Cleft Width**
- Among patients with alveolar clefts, increasing
- bony width was associated with worse columellar
- angle, nostril height ratio, and nostril width ratio
- before surgery (0.61, 0.70, and 0.34, respectively).
- Following surgery, the association persisted immediately
- postoperatively (0.31) and at later followup
- (0.59).
- Comment: *width is really important;the wide ones are very hard to treat*

Childrens Hospital MA Discussions

- Whereas primary rhinoplasty generally entails
- nasal tip dissection with or without suturing of tip
- cartilages, we describe an alternate approach that
- focuses on the foundation to correct the nose. It
- follows principles of wide surgical release, component
- reconstruction, and attention to anatomical
- subunits As such, the cutaneous nasal sill, muscle, septum, floor, sidewall, and tipcartilages should be considered individually.. provided an opportunity
- to determine nasal changes produced by correcting
- the foundation, without nasal tip correction…
- *comment:* *routine everyday procedure with a hypothesis which is being studied*

- considerable correction
- of nasal form can be achieved by means
- of septum, floor, and sidewall correction, before
- muscle and skin closure, and without any dissection
- of the tip…
- *comment:* *routine procedure, plus minus tip modifications..many use different variations wthout giving it exotic names*

- Septal deviation was almost universal (even for incomplete clefts); and septal repositioning produced considerable changes... subperiosteal approach that avoids delamination of the cartilage...
- comment: *routine*
- There is a notion that the caudal septum can dislocate onto the noncleft side and that septal reposition reduces the dislocation... he will show this.. septoplasty
- Long term studies alone will show this.. septoplasty "dislocates" the septum and places it in a nonanatomical position, at the midline of the face.
- The long-term consequences of this surgical dislocation is unknown; however, studies thus far suggest that there is no impact on growth
- turbinate flap provides broad robust tissue, and removal of the underlying bone potentially alleviates obstruction of a narrowed nasal airway:

- However, the flap is difficult to access if there is no cleft in the palate through which instruments can pass to make the posterior incision: In addition, because of its base along the piriform margin, the posterior extent of nasal floor closure is limited to a level anterior to the lesser segment alveolus.

- The L-flap is always available, regardless of cleft type, and can provide a continuous layer of closure with additional elevation of nasal mucoperiosteum. Lateral wall advancement provides broad robust tissue, avoids obliteration of normal anatomy, and replaces tissues in kind: Perhaps the greatest advantage is that it allows continuous posterior nasal floor closure beyond the alveolar ridge...
- comment: *A rerun on Noordhoff over many years ad lib*

Childrens Hospital MA Discussions
Childrens Hospital MA Discussions

- Lower lateral cartilage dissection is often considered
- the sine qua non of primary cleft rhinoplasty.
- Our report is unique in that none of the
- subjects underwent such dissection.. *comment:* *reinventions will go on till the rapture*

- Even with primary nasal tip dissection,
- secondary correction is undertaken in 35
- to 70 percent of patients,3–7 as

  there is a "perverse

- tendency for the genu to slump with time
- *comment:*
- *comment:* *why Tajima is not an absolute solution ,but a temporary measure*

59

Childrens Hospital MA Discussions

- By preserving tissue planes of the nasal tip, surgery may be facilitated, and the ultimate outcome may be improved. Future assessment at maturity is
- paramount.
- *Comment:* opinions vary on this gentle dissection using fine scissors

    preserve tissue quite well

- we found that both alar
- base and lip commissures changed with surgery
- and thus the ratio did not change. Over the course
- of several years, the commissures widen and the ratio increases.
- *Comment:* useful studies which you have done so many times..

Childrens Hospital MA Discussions

- there is currently no consensus on the
- best way to assess outcome of nasal reconstruction.
- We used traditional anthropometric measurements
- so that comparison can be made to other
- studies…
- *comment:* the best there is

today…but useful

- Of 102 patients, five underwent lip
- taping and 15 underwent

nasoalveolar molding…

- *comment:* NAM vs no NAM..useful to know long term outcomes across countries

- Significant correction of the unilateral cleft lip
- nasal deformity can be achieved by correction of septum,
- floor, and sidewall, without nasal tip dissection…Changes in objective measures of three-dimensional
- form approached those of age-matched controls
- and persisted at 5 years of age. Preservation of tissue
- planes may allow for easier or better secondary revision,
- if necessary.
- Comment: *useful armamentarium used globally*

- Significant correction of the unilateral cleft lip
- nasal deformity can be achieved by correction of septum,
- jewall, without nasal tip dissection…Changes in objective three-dimensional
- ched those of age-matched controls
- d at 5 years of age. Preservation of tissue
- allow for easier or better secondary revision,

- Dear Bona,
- I very much enjoyed your dissection and comments on the Tse MS.
- I smiled and agreed with most of your responses.
- I must admit, I don't see the problem addressed by the L-flap (Millard's contribution, not Noordhoff); inferior turbinate flap or the new lateral vestibular flap: I find once: elevated; there is an excess of lateral vestibular (mucoperiosteal) lining:
- Can you direct me to the best illustration of the CGMC (Noordho inferior turbinate flap?
- I hope we are on the same page?
- John B M

- Dear Bona,
- I very much enjoyed your
- Tse MS.
- I smiled and agreed with
- responses.
- I must admit, I don't see t
- (Millard's contribution, no
- the new lateral vestibular
- excess of lateral vestibula
- Can you direct me to the
- inferior turbinate flap?
- I hope we are on the sam
- John B M

Dear John,

Thank you for your mail. Yes, I believe there is no solid take-home message in the paper that helps us improve any existing technique or outcome.

I agree with you completely on the floor of nose ideas. There is often excess tissue, depending on the width of the cleft.

As for the Noordhoff technique on the ITF flap, I assisted both P Chen and Lo on their modifications. The results are comparable, no matter which modification is used.

It is not always easy to understand the movements of the flap. This is true, especially for newcomers. So I came up with a simple analogy of the pear which I attach here. I use the ITF pics from Noordhoff's great book on UCL cheiloplasty for personal study and also to share with my friends who are new to it.

best,

Bona

Putting the three flaps together to reconstruct the floor of nose using the analogy of a pear
JOUR IDEA @ Room 643 CGMH

imagine the inferior turbinate is like a pear handing inside the nostril tree

90 degrees movement of pear

Inferior turbinate mucosa

alar Right

Pyriform rim

Noordhoff point

Pyriform rim edge

superior part

inferior part

medial part

L flap   CM flap   R

- The incisional approach to the inferior pole of the inferior turbinate flap is easy, trace along the Noordhoff point and incise between skin and mucosa up the vestibule skin, cut along the inferior part of the turbinate, then follow the pear all around and connect to the superior pole

- A small transverse stab between the lower lateral cartilages is the superior entry point

- Connect the pear and after reducing the bone to prevent buckling of the flap, rotate it down by 90 degrees

- The superior pole edge is fixed to the pyriform edge to provide lining for the nose

- The inferior edge joins the L flap and is sutured as a turn over flap to the turned over CM flap

- This completes the floor of nose correction

14: Pictures and Comments :

1.Before and after the Tajima procedure and 3D printed nasal conformers

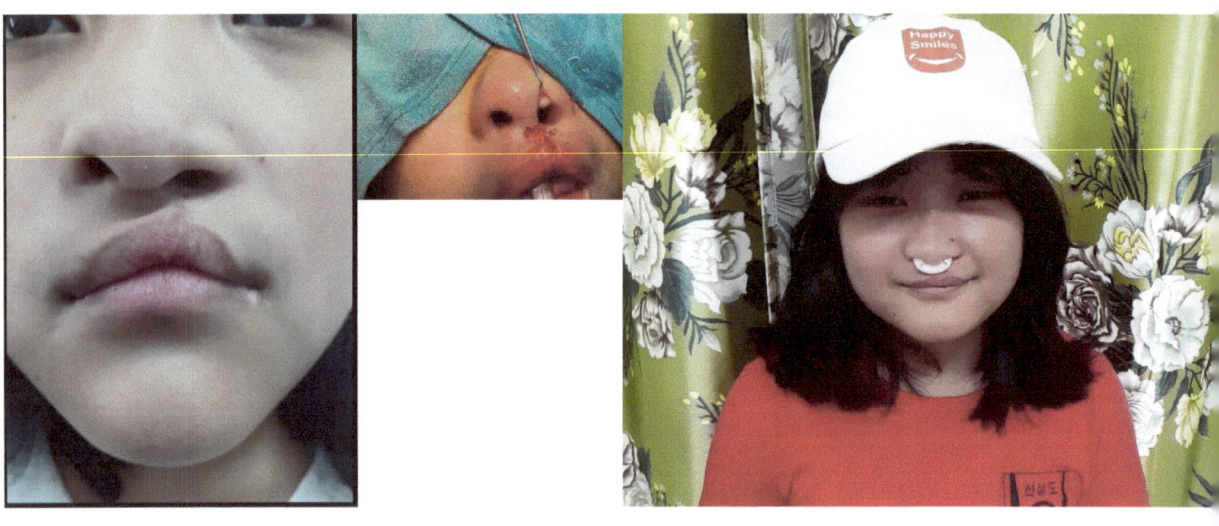

2.Child with Tessier 7 cleft before and

after (Mulliken's online advice)

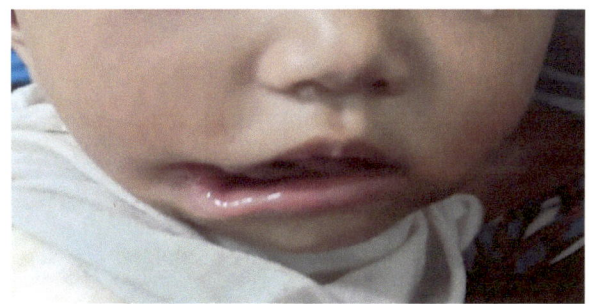 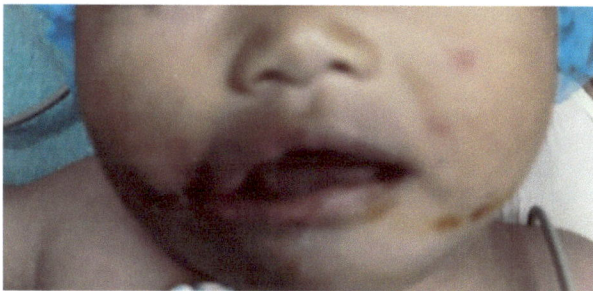

4. Happy Smiles @ CIHSR Surgery
4. Happy Smiles @ CIHSR Surgery
(post op nasal floor infection leading to slight deformity of left nose)
(post op nasal floor infection leading to slight deformity of left nose)

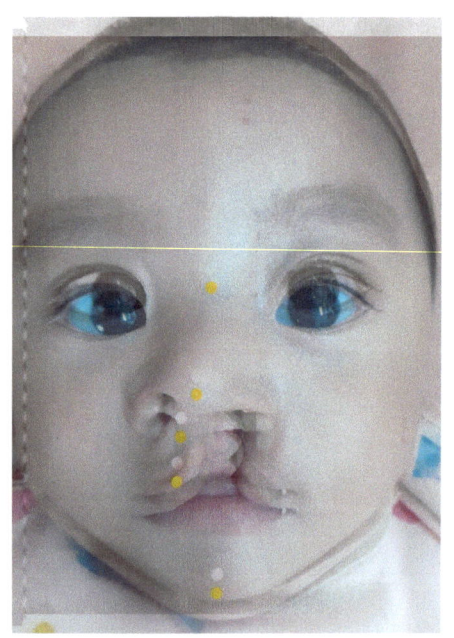

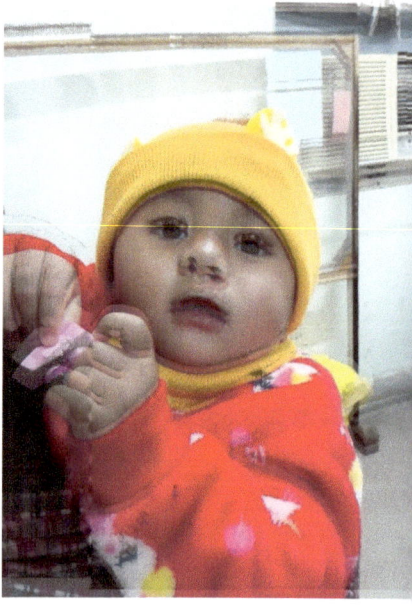

5: Happy Smiles @ CIHSR Surgery for severe bilateral cleft lip deformity,and the use of our 3 D nasal conformers

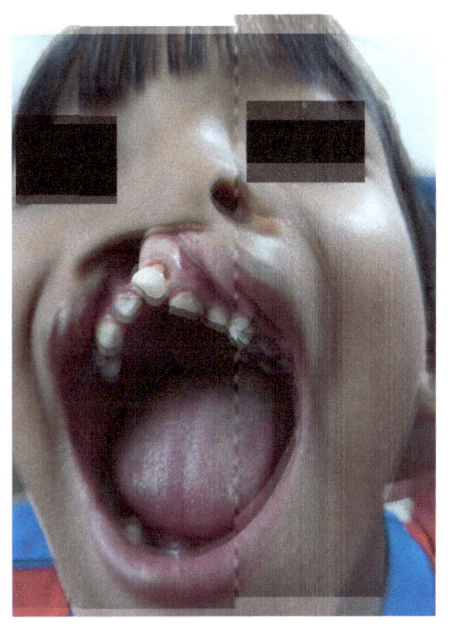

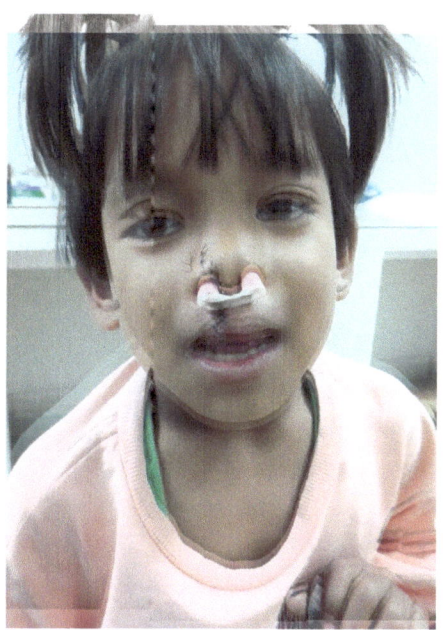

6. Happy Smiles @ CIHSR Surgery , unilateral cleft lip complete

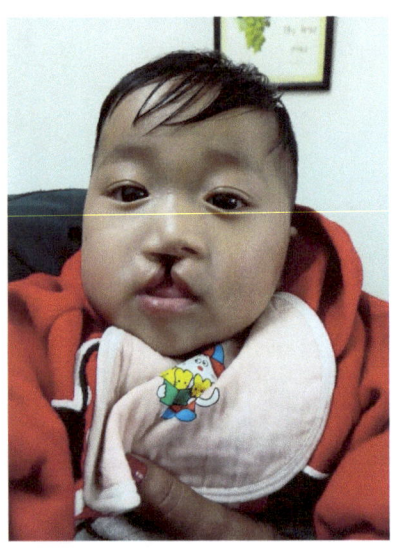
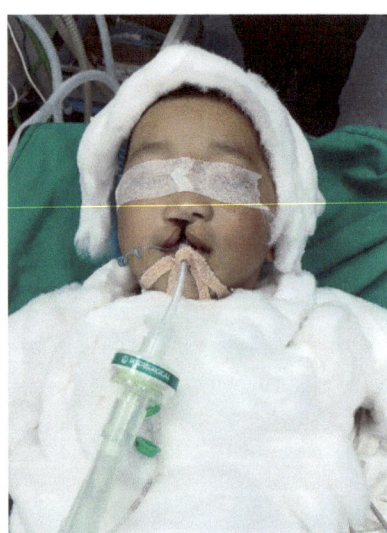
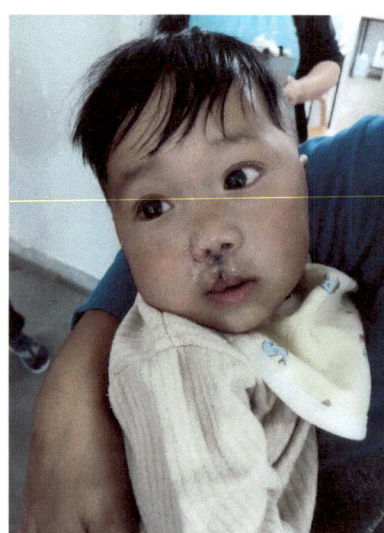

7. Happy Smiles @ CIHSR Surgery, revision of maladjusted left cleft lip and nose

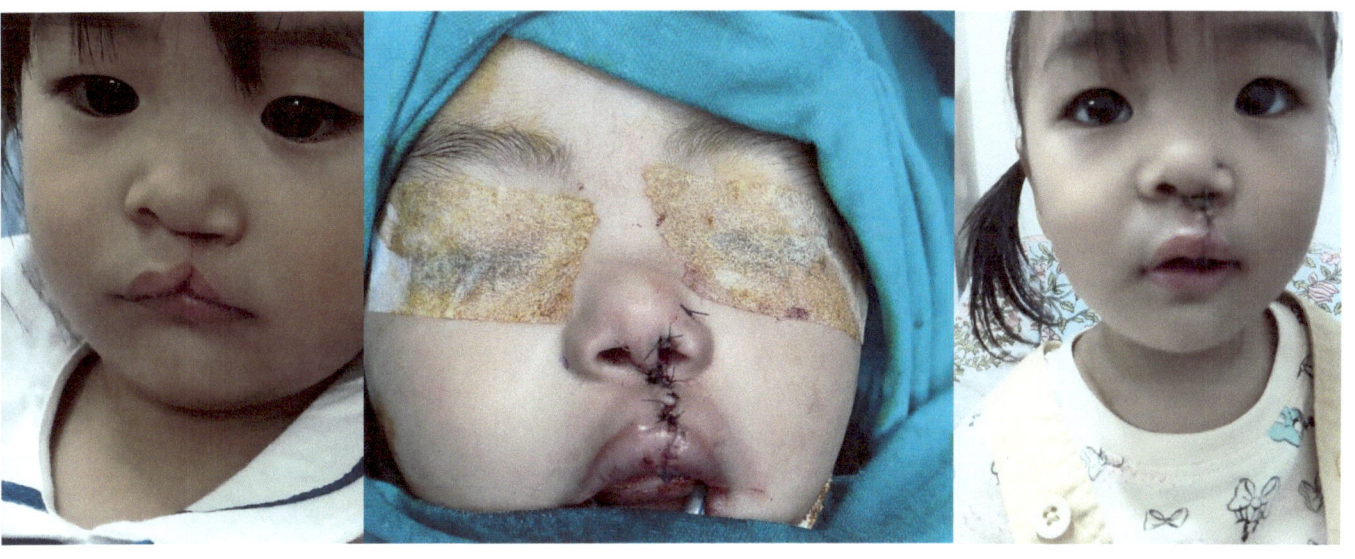

8. Modification in very difficult cleft, First sponsored patient Najuna @ CIHSR done by Dr. Temsula and team@ Happy Smiles

Comment: "Good Job" Prof L J Lo, Chang Gung Craniofacial Centre Taipei

8: Modification in very difficult cleft, First sponsored patient Najuna @ CIHSR done by Dr. Temsula and team@ Happy Smiles

Comment: "Good Job" Prof L J Lo, Chang Gung Craniofacial Centre Taipei

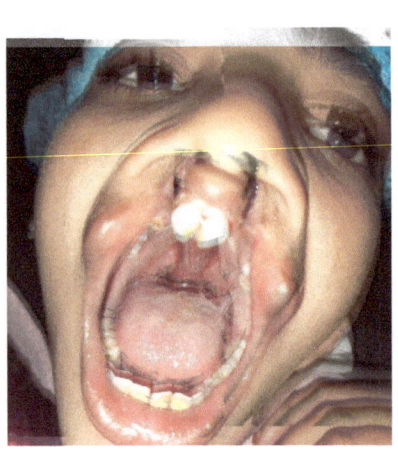
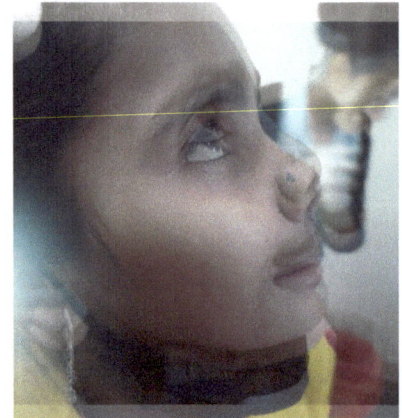
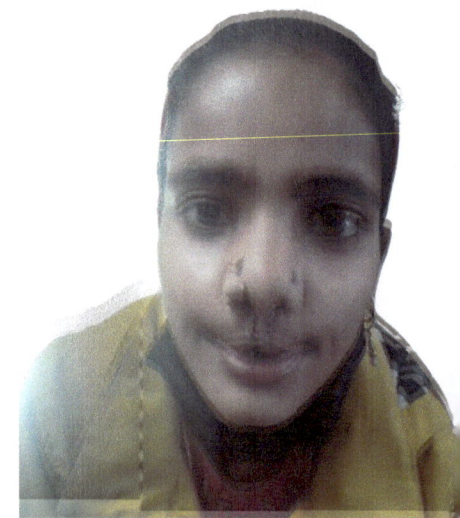

8: Post trauma patient with lip deformity, Ho Chi Minh City, Vietnam Designing a cleft lip to correct a bad scar
9: Post trauma patient with lip deformity, Ho Chi Minh City, Vietnam Designing a cleft lip to correct a bad scar

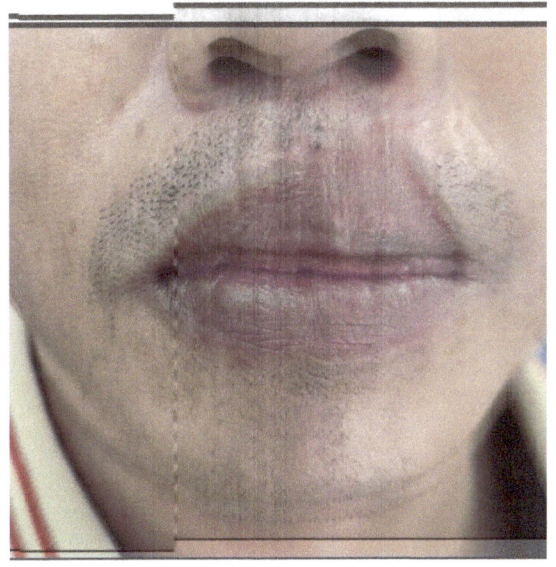
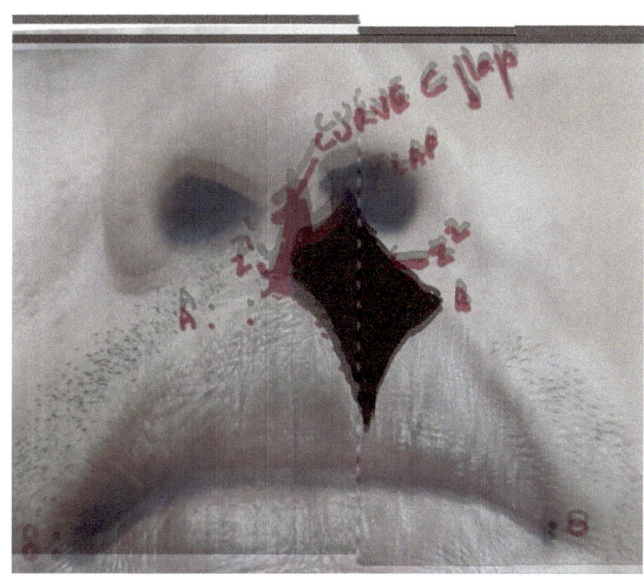

Successful cleft lip transposition at OMS Hospital, Ho Chi Minh City, Vietnam last week comment:
" John B Mulliken, Childrens MA ..Great result on the post-traumatic scar to CL transposition"

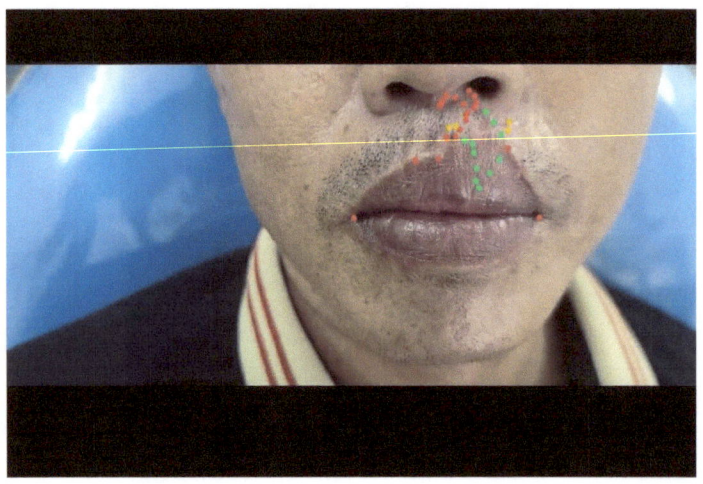
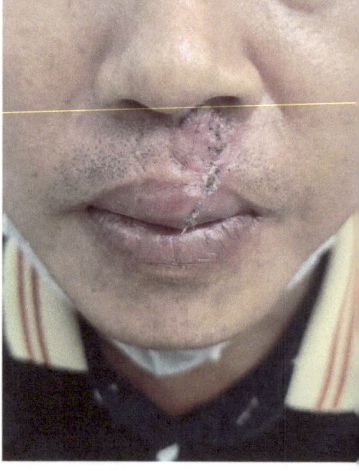

10.   A Happy Smile Family from Assam, after correction of a bilateral asymmetric cleft lip

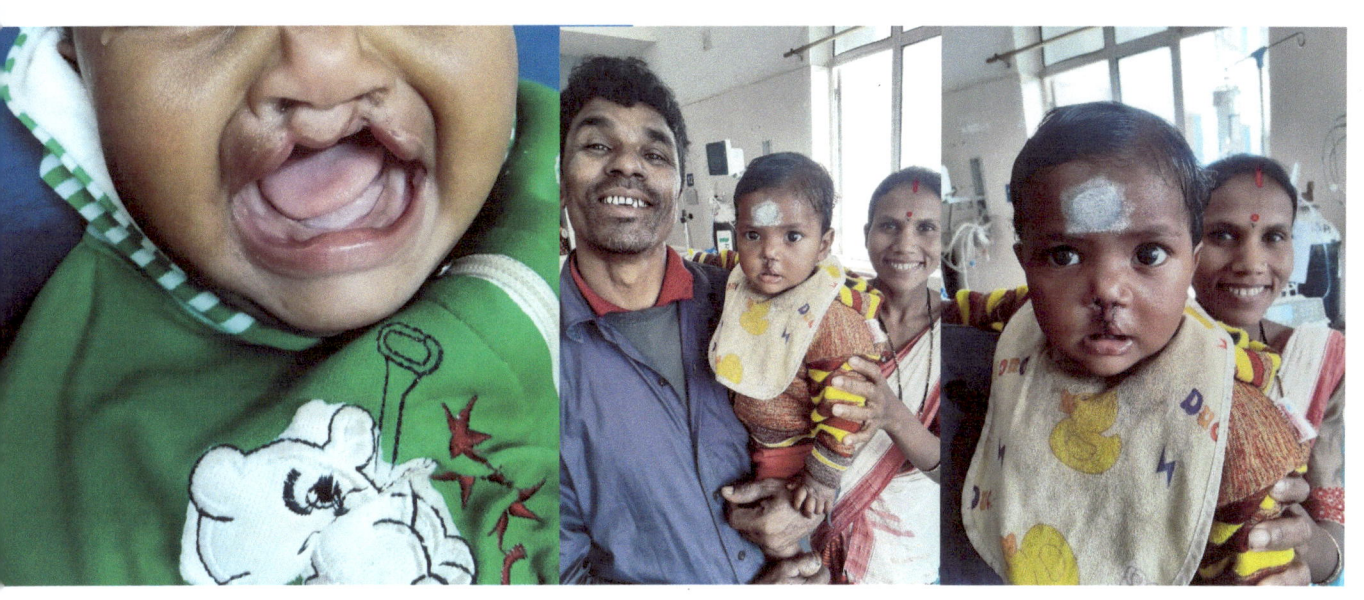

11. Unilateral complete Cleft lip in a child 11 months old
11. Unilateral complete Cleft lip in a child 11 months old

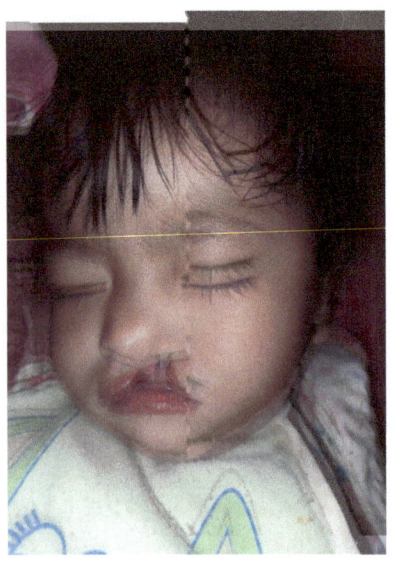
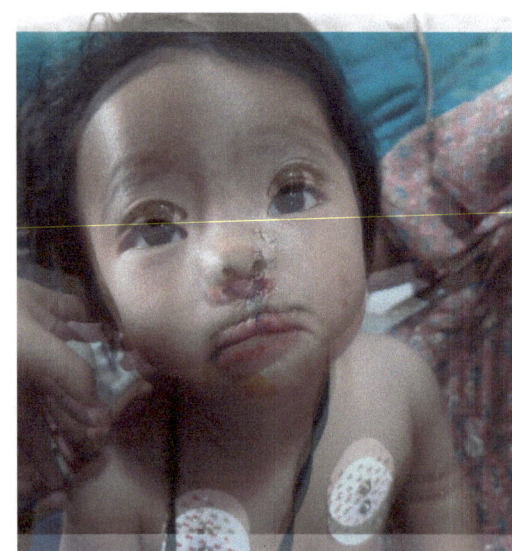
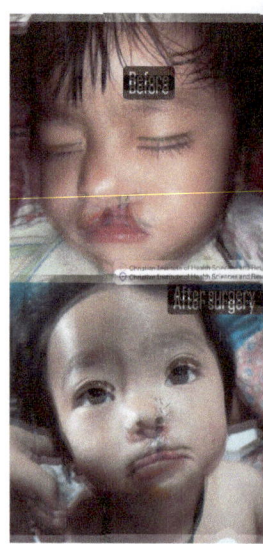

12. Happy Smiles @ CIHSR Surgery 2023, unilateral cleft lip
12. Happy Smiles @ CIHSR Surgery 2023, unilateral cleft lip

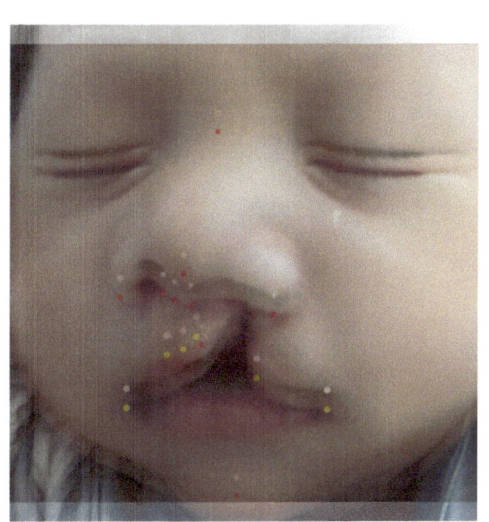

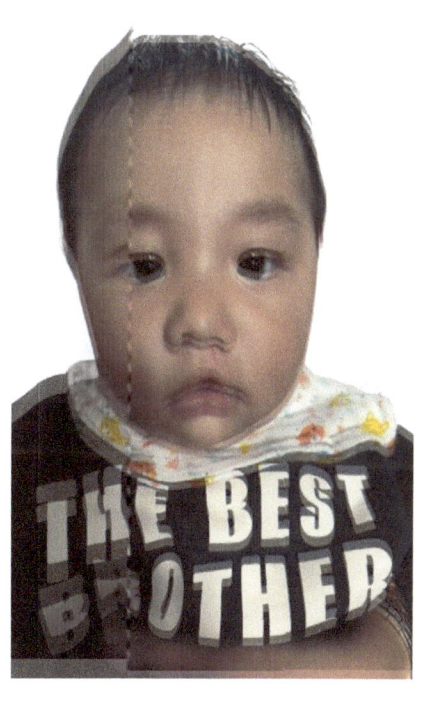

13. Microform cleft lip in a baby- And remember to smile always!

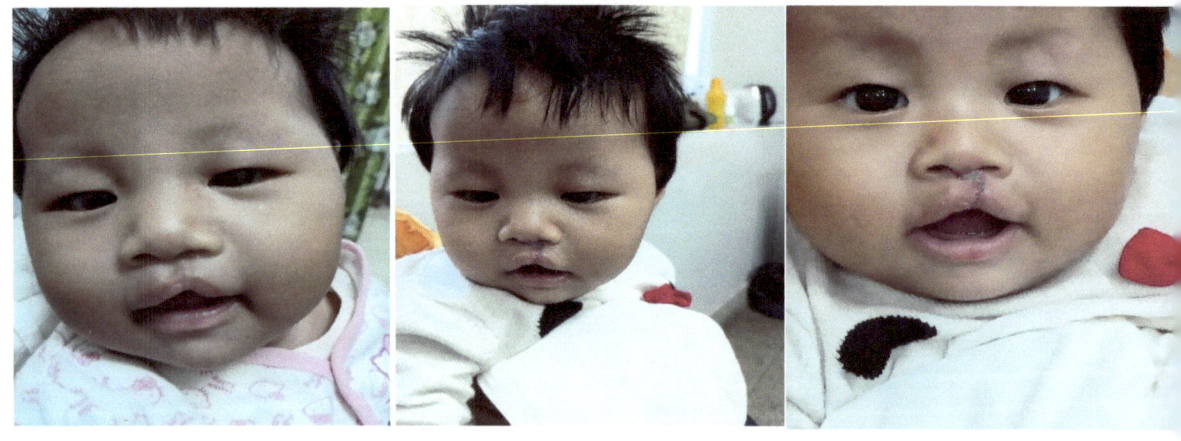

14: unilateral cleft lip repair : From the cradle to the last crinkle

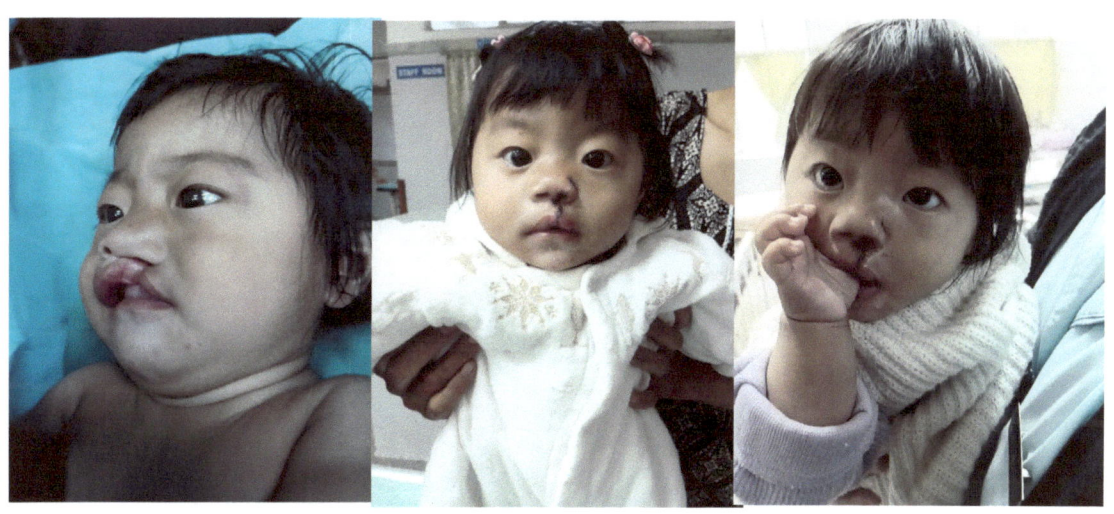

15.Palatoplasty in Latecomers using saline hydrodissection1:500,00 adr and button hole incisions to
medialize flaps without tension Year 2003 Yemen

15.Palatoplasty in Latecomers using saline hydrodissection1:500,00 adr and button hole incisions to
medialize flaps without tension Year 2003 Yemen

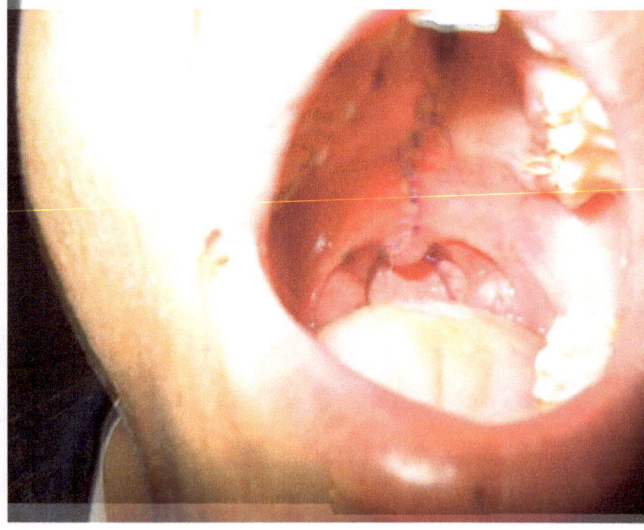

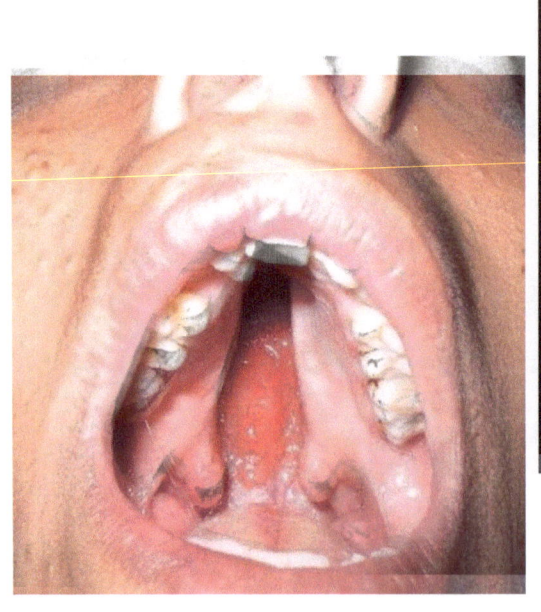

16.Saline hydro dissection with significant gap reduction and minimal bleeding
16.Saline hydro dissection with significant gap reduction and minimal bleeding
The Happy Smiles-CIHSR modified technique
The Happy Smiles-CIHSR modified technique

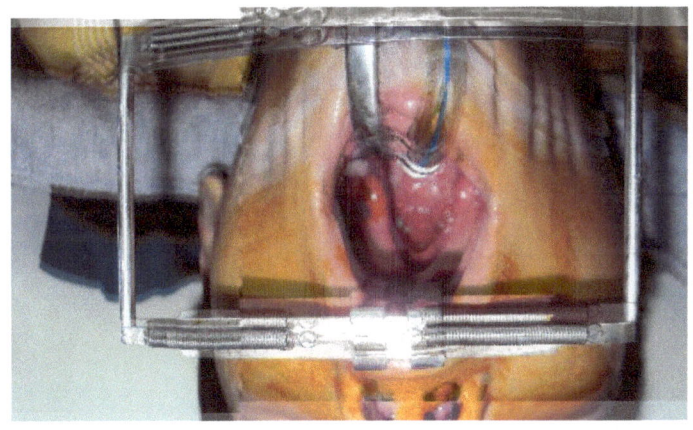

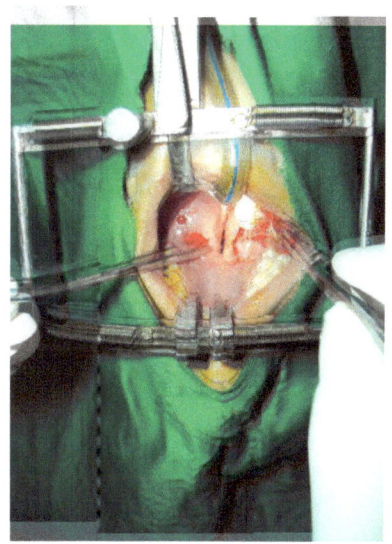

16.Levator retro positioning 7-10 mm, and tension free closure

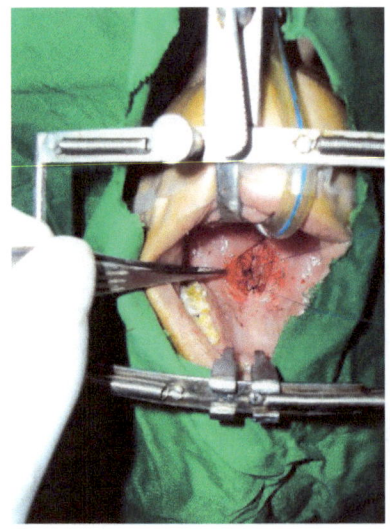 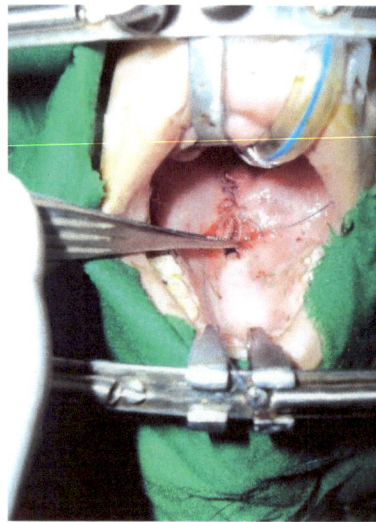

17. The Future of cleft lip surgery

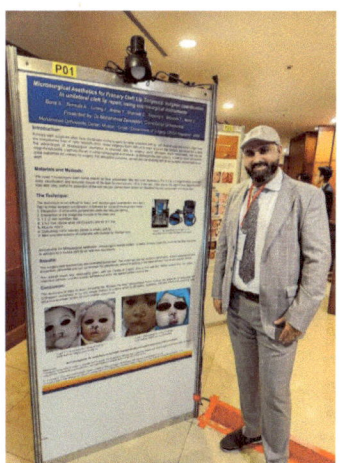

ORIGINAL POSTER CONCEPT

2023 APCA, APCLPC & CHANG GUNG FORUM
THE 13TH BIENNIAL CONGRESS OF ASIAN PACIFIC
CRANIOFACIAL ASSOCIATION
THE 10TH ASIAN PACIFIC CLEFT LIP-PALATE & CRANIOFACIAL
CONGRESS
THE 9TH INTERNATIONAL WORKSHOP ON SURGERY-FIRST
ORTHOGNATHIC SURGERY
THE GRAND HOTEL, TAIPEI, TAIWAN
NOVEMBER 6~8, 2023

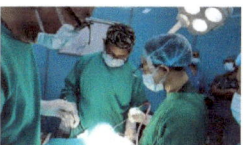

Microsurgical Aesthetics for Primary Cleft Lip Surgeons: surgeon
coordination in unilateral cleft lip repair, using microsurgical instruments
Bona S , Temsula A, Lurong I, Aremo Y,Shamuel G,Tiapong A,Wonashi
T,Mohd Z

Microsurgical Aesthetic Smiles @ Dept of Surgery, CIHSR Nagaland/MOC
Muscat Oman

Microsurgical Aesthetics for Primary Cleft Lip Surgeons: surgeon coordination in unilateral cleft lip repair, using microsurgical instruments

Bona S. , Temsula A. , Lurong I. , Aremo Y. , Shamuel G. , Tiapong A. ,Wonashi T. , Mohd Z.

Presented by: Dr Mohammad Zeinalddin, Craniofacial Orthodontist

Mohammad Orthodontic Center, Muscat - Oman / Department of Surgery, CIHSR Nagaland - India

Introduction:

Primary cleft surgeons often face challenges during surgery for wider unilateral cleft lip, with floor of nose deformities. Apart from the complicated floor of nose reconstruction, newer surgeons find it difficult to make accurate flap designs. We would like to post the advantages of microsurgical aesthetics in nuanced cleft lip surgery, using affordable micro instruments and clip on magnifiers/loupes. Learning the art of using microsurgical instruments, and through-the-loop suturing, in cleft lip repair can provide good outcomes for primary lip surgery. For simulation purposes, we will also be studying cleft lip using digital microscopes in our work.

Materials and Methods:

We used microsurgery instruments mainly for finer procedures, after the main dissections.The 2.5 to 3.5 magnification provided easy visualization and accurate closure of the flaps for mucosa and 1.5 to 2 mm skin z flap above the Cupid's bow. Magnification was also very useful for dissection of the sub reticular dermis plane where we identified the pars peripheralis and marginalis.

The Technique:

The technique is not difficult to learn, and requires good coordination as a team.
Two to three surgeon coordination is followed for some of the important steps[1]:
1. Dissection of orbicularis peripheralis under the reticular dermis,
2. Dissection of the marginalis muscle at the lower end.
3. 1.5 –2 mm vermilion flap,
4. 1.5-2 mm above white roll (Cupid's), and tip of C flap
5. Muscle mini z
6. Debulking minor salivary glands in a fatty cleft lip
7. Mini eversion sutures of marginalis and mucosa for Parisian pout

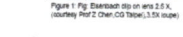

Figure 1: Fig. Eisenbach clip on lens 2.5 X,
(courtesy Prof Z Chen,CG Taipei),3.5X loupe)

Instruments for Microsurgical Aesthetics : microsurgical needle holders, scissors, forceps, small skin hooks for the finer dissection, in addition to a routine cleft lip set with fine instruments

Results:

The surgery was successfully demonstrated to trainees[2]. The challenge was two surgeon coordination, which is essential for micro dissection, otherwise one can cut through the peripheralis instead of staying in the plane between muscle and reticular dermis.

The overall result was reasonably good, with the Centre of Cupid's bow in line with the midline vertical from the nasion to pogonion vertical, and the nostrils symmetrical within the medial canthal vertical line.

Conclusion:

The technique is easy to learn, including the "through the loop" microsurgical suture method. We would like to encourage our colleagues elsewhere, to try this simple method of surgery which is affordable, applicable, and cost effective for providing more attractive aesthetic smiles for cleft children everywhere

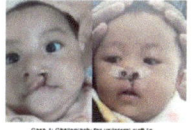
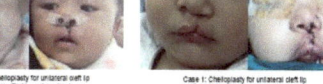

Case 1: Cheiloplasty for unilateral cleft lip
(Left, before), (Right, post op day 1)

Case 1: Cheiloplasty for unilateral cleft lip
(Left, before), (Right, post op immediate)

Acknowledgments: We would like to thank CIHSR , Nagaland and Muscat teams for preparation of this presentation

References:
1. Anatomy of the KISS Principle for Trainee Cleft Surgeons: The Quest for a Cleft Aesthetic Code of the Philtrum and Median Tubercle in Unilateral Cleft Lip Surgery using Strictly Anatomical Concepts Bona L, The Cleft Palate-Craniofacial Journal 2020, Vol. 57(4)I: 1-143

2. "Learning to Crack the Cleft Aesthetic Code in Unilateral Cleft Lip Surgery by Younger Cleft Trainees: Using Nuances and the Innovative Taipei Pear Analogy for Inferior Turbinate-flap Floor of Nose Reconstruction", Bona L,Mohd Z et al. Acta Scientific Paediatrics 3.3 (2020): 10-16

18.Comments and advice from mentors
18.Comments and advice from mentors

Yeap CL Mount Elizabeth Plastic Surgery ,Orchard Road Singapore
Yeap CL Mount Elizabeth Plastic Surgery ,Orchard Road Singapore

http://www.dryeapplasticsurgery.sg/

"Dear Bona Thank you so much for your wonderful work inspired by our Almighty God:
"Dear Bona Thank you so much for your wonderful work inspired by our
Keep sharing your blessings with the cleft patients and surgeons."
Keep sharing your blessings with the cleft patients and surgeons."

Yeap:
Yeap:
Farrer Park Hospital
Farrer Park Hospital
Singapore
Singapore

Acknowledgments:
Acknowledgments:

"Some of our best cosmetic techniques were learnt from

Yeap over nearly ten years."

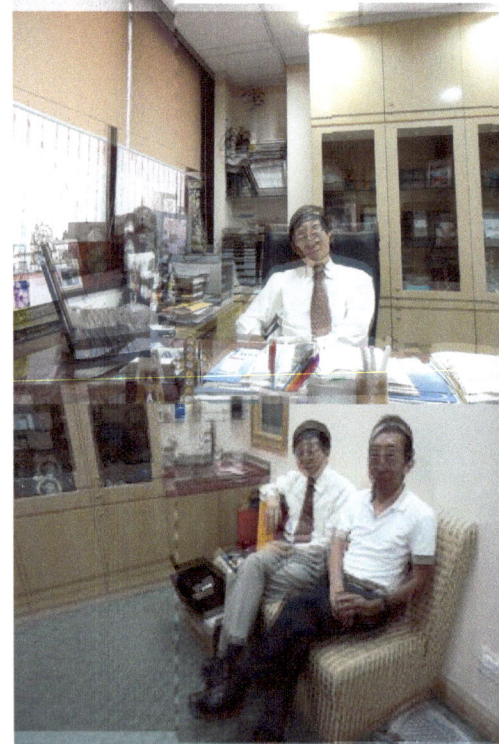

19. Comments and advice from mentors : Childrens,MA .

From 2008 July till date, over 17 years, John has patiently mentored our group in state of the art advances of cleft lip and palate surgery:

- John B Mulliken ,Childrens MA

Bona,

Comments on anthropometry: Good question: Someday, I hope to analyze the Kriens and Mulliken types of bilateral cleft revision. Suggest you re-read the Kim and Mulliken paper on long-term anthropometry of BCCL. The curves tell you how the critical dimensions change in time—these should help you in designing the repair. Note how the transverse dimensions widen; height of median tubercle lags; etc.

Comment on wrong lip repair techniques: (bccl secondary) Bona,

Agree. These BCCL repairs are from the 19th and early 20th century.

John

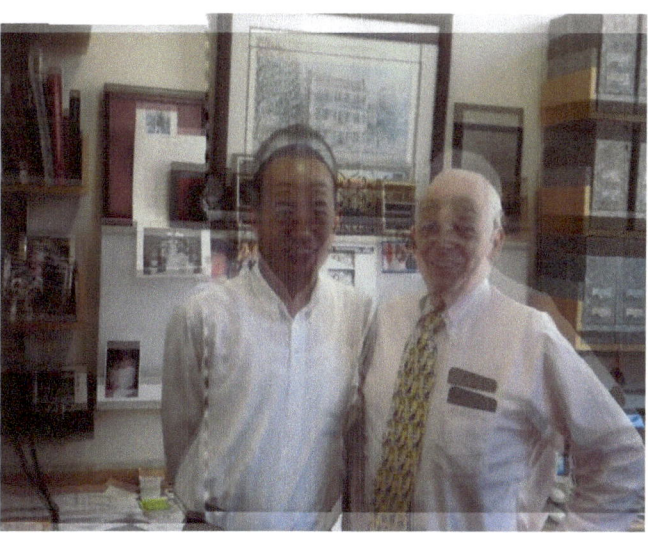

20.With Philip Chen of Chang Gung Craniofacial Taipei 2006

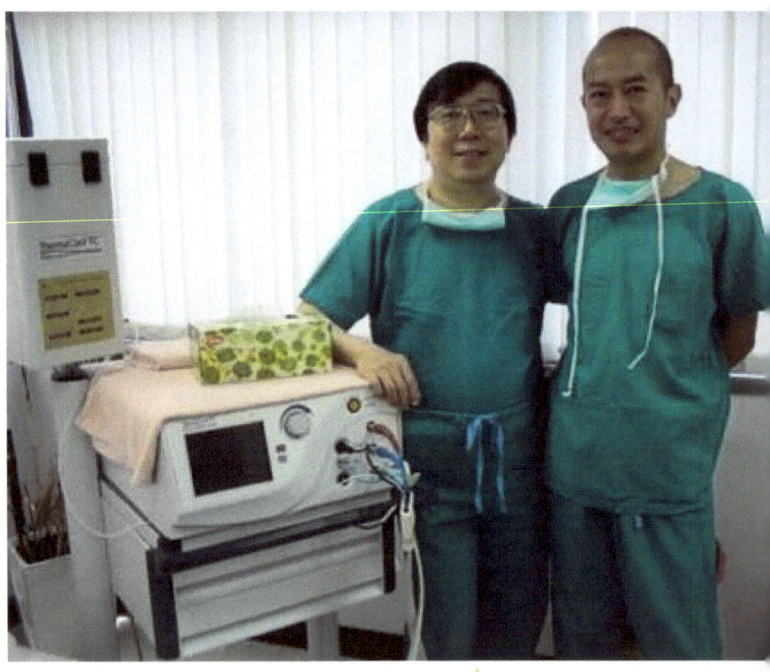

21: Happy Smiles for cleft lip and palate children

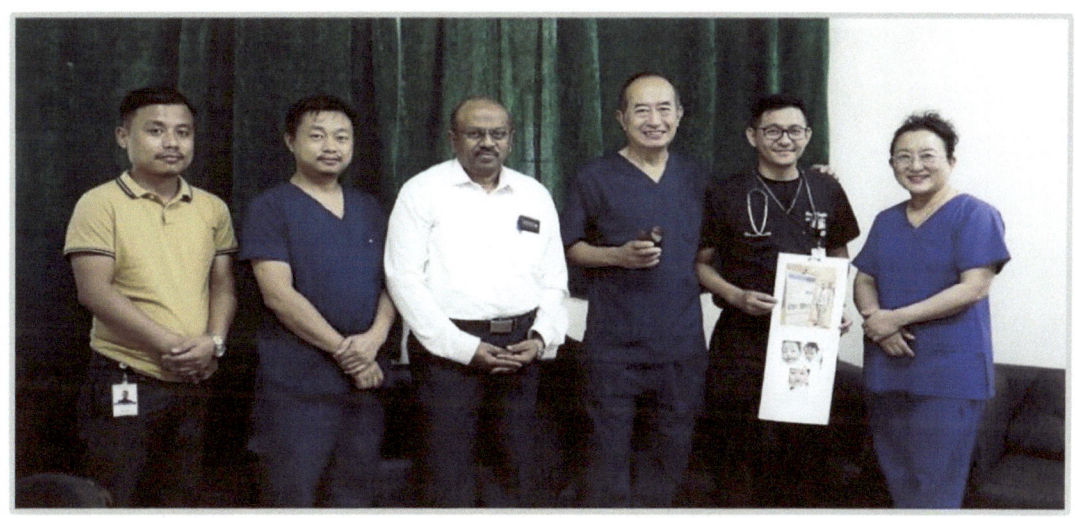

The Nitty Gritty Smile Team

22.Happy Smiles @ Dept. of Surgery CIHS
22.Happy Smiles @ Dept. of Surgery CIHSR

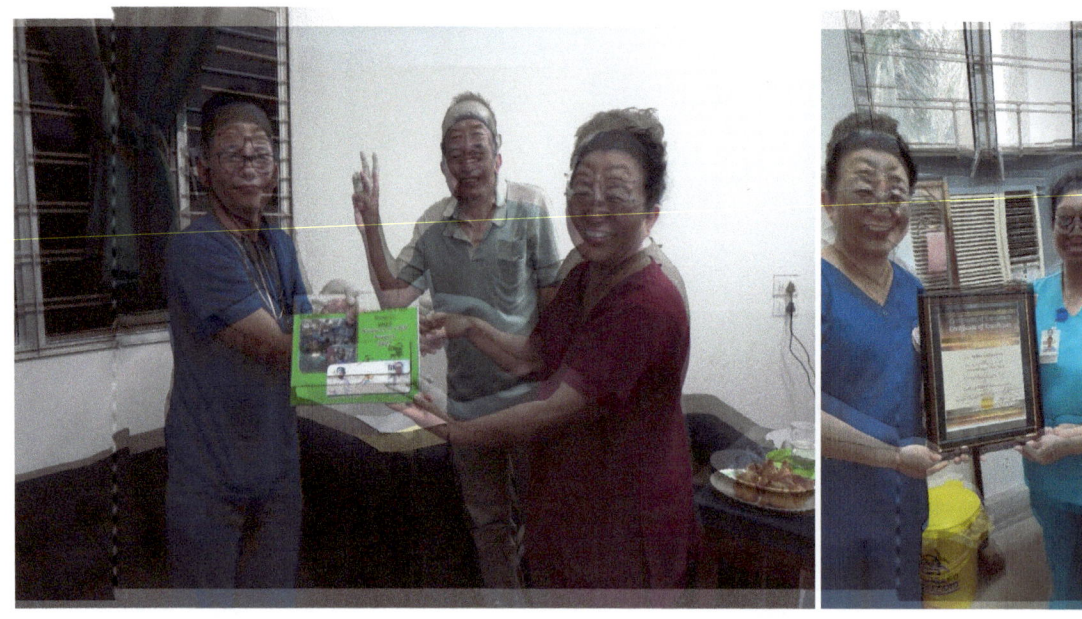

23.Arabic, Russian and English Version by Drs. Mohd and Bona
23.Arabic, Russian and English Version by Drs. Mohd and Bona

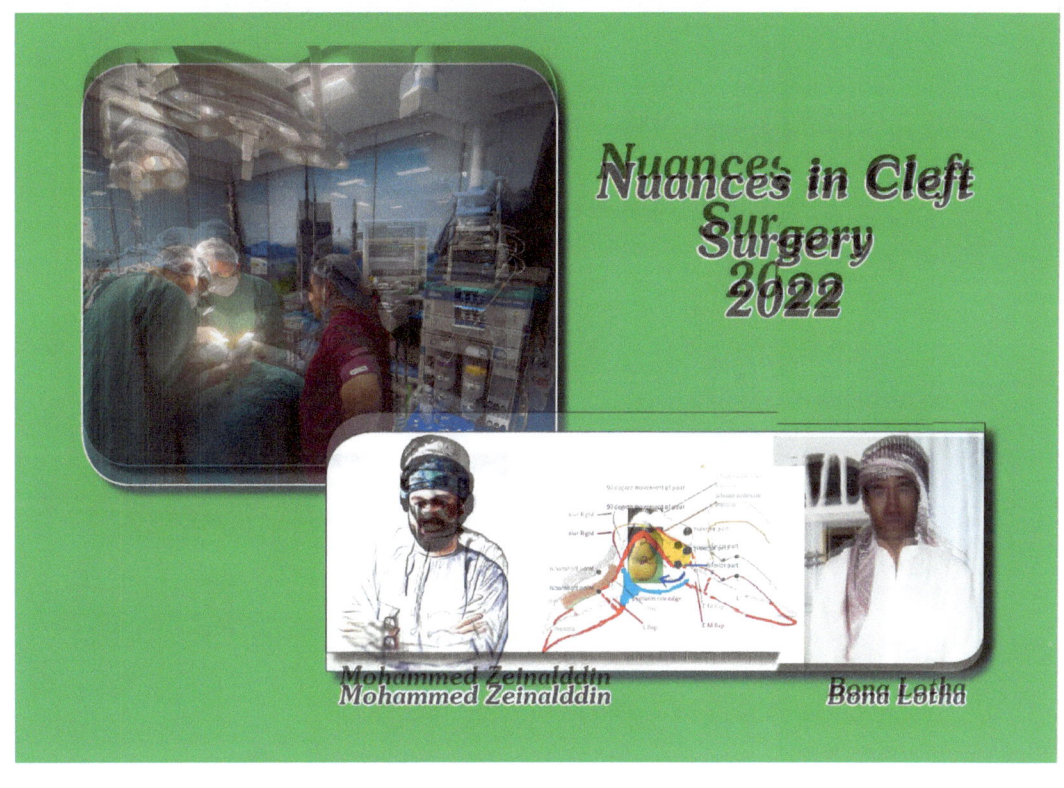

24.Shukran Chopsticks!

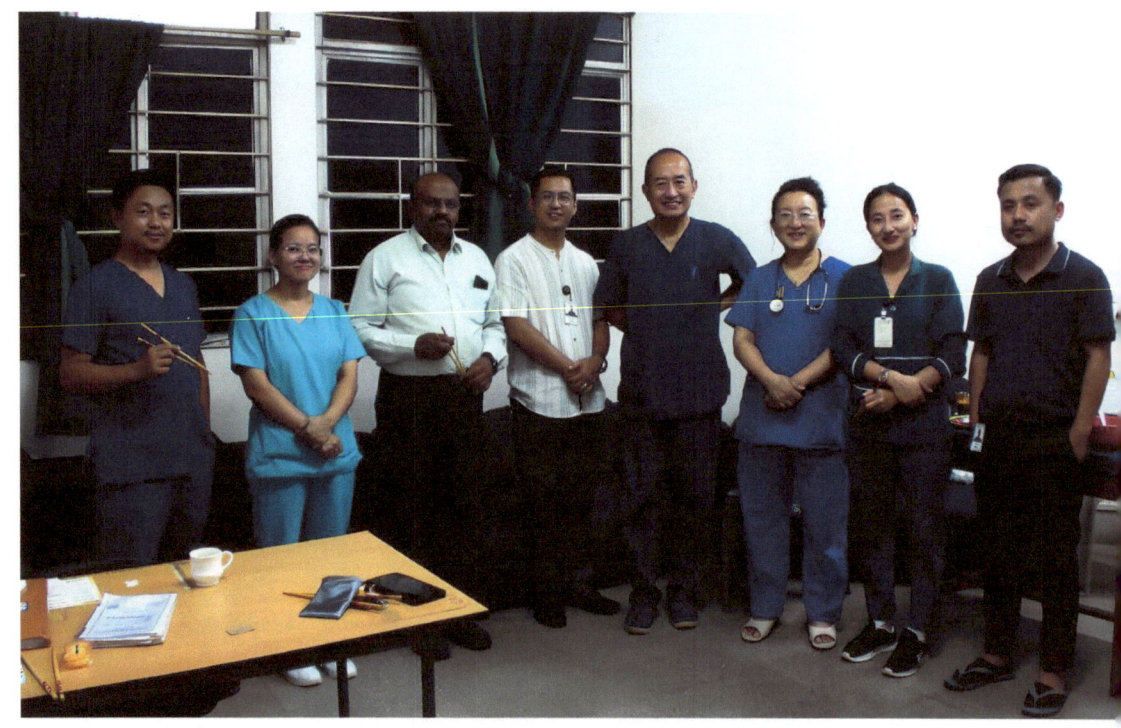

Happy
Smiles

www.ingramcontent.com/pod-product-compliance
Lightning Source LLC
Chambersburg PA
CBHW051949210526
45474CB00003B/64